Brain Gym®

Teacher's Edition
Revised

The companion guide to the *Brain Gym* book, for parents, educators, and all others interested in the relationship between movement and whole-brain learning

Paul E. Dennison, Ph.D.

Gail E. Dennison

Illustrated by Gail E. Dennison

Edu-Kinesthetics, Inc.
Ventura, California

The Edu-Kinesthetics Learning-Through-Movement Series:

Edu-K for Kids
Brain Gym®
Brain Gym® Teacher's Edition

ISBN 0-942143-02-7

Acknowledgments

The authors wish to recognize the many hundreds of individuals who have brought Brain Gym® to their students, schools, and communities. The *Brain Gym* book is used throughout the English-speaking world, including the United States, Canada, the United Kingdom, Australia, and New Zealand, and has been translated into nine languages. This *Teacher's Edition* was created out of many individuals' shared belief that "movement is the door to learning."

Special thanks

to Azasha Joy Lindsey, who first believed in networking Brain Gym information

to Gabrell Carroll, Rose Harrow, and George and Colleen Gardner, who live Brain Gym and teach it at all levels

to Guruchiter Kaur Khalsa and Josie Sifft, who completed the first experimental research studies which correlated Brain Gym movements and improved performance

to Nancy Kaplan Marshall, who first made us aware of the need for a handbook for teachers

to Carla Hannaford, who encouraged us to write a program for educators, and who offered the innovation of Quadroodle Doodles

to Sandra Hinsley, who draws out the best from her students with Brain Gym movements, and who created the 3-D Breathing variation of Belly Breathing

to Dr. Byung Kyu Park, for his useful variation on Belly Breathing

to Dorothy H. L. Carroll, whose commitment to bring Brain Gym to professional educators inspired us to create this handbook

to Sarab Atma Kaur for her dedicated typing and proofreading of the original manuscript

to Lark Carroll for her enthusiastic editing and suggestions

to Susan Latham, whose movement with her students is an inspiration to us all

to Sonia Nordenson and Jari Chevalier for their editing and proofreading of this most recent, revised edition

For Your Information

The movements and activities described in this book are solely for educational use. The authors and Edu-Kinesthetics, Inc., do not intend to present any part of this work as a diagnosis or prescription for any ailment of any reader or student, nor are they responsible for anyone misrepresenting this program by such claim.

It is recommended that you consult your medical professional before beginning any movement program.

When starting an exercise program, it is important to remember that skills should be built up gradually, over time. All of these exercises are intended to be easy and comfortable to perform at all times.

This self-help program will complement, support, and enhance your current medical or educational program, whether it be with a medical doctor, a chiropractor, a behavioral optometrist, or an educational therapist.

To learn more about the Brain Gym program, write to:

The Educational Kinesiology Foundation
P.O. Box 3396, Ventura, CA 93006
or call (800) 356-2109.

Table of Contents

About the Authors

Paul E. Dennison, Ph.D., has been an educator for all of his professional life. He is the creator of the Edu-Kinesthetics and Brain Gym processes, and a pioneer in applied brain research. His discoveries are based upon an understanding of the interdependence of physical development, language acquisition, and academic achievement. This perspective grew out of his background in curriculum development and experimental psychology at the University of Southern California, where he was granted a Doctorate in Education for his research in beginning reading achievement and its relationship to thinking. For nineteen years, Dr. Dennison served as director of the Valley Remedial Group Learning Centers in Southern California, helping children and adults turn their difficulties into successful growth. He is the author of twelve books and manuals, including *Switching On: A Guide to Edu-Kinesthetics*.

Gail E. Dennison is the co-author with her husband, Dr. Dennison, of the Edu-Kinesthetics series of books and manuals. The simple illustrations in the Edu-K books speak of her love of children and movement. As a dancer, she has brought grace and focus to the Brain Gym® activities. Gail has a varied background in the teaching of brain integration, including ten years' experience as a Touch for Health instructor. Gail's interest in perception and developmental skills comes through in the Edu-K vision courses. She developed the *Visioncircles* course and the *Vision Gym*™ movements, in which rhythm, color, and form provide the basis for experiences that offer visual and perceptual growth. Gail is the creator of the *Brain Gym Journal*, and heads the publication committee for the Educational Kinesiology Foundation.

A Message to Parents and Educators

Brain Gym® is a series of simple and enjoyable movements that we use with our students in Educational Kinesiology (Edu-K) to enhance their experience of whole-brain learning. These activities make all types of learning easier, and are especially effective with academic skills. The word education comes from the Latin word *educare*, which means "to draw out." Kinesiology, derived from the Greek root *kinesis*, means "motion," and is the study of the movement of the human body. Educational Kinesiology is a system for empowering learners of any age by using movement activities to draw out hidden potential and make it readily available.

Traditionally, educators have addressed failure by devising programs to better motivate, entice, reinforce, drill, and "stamp in" learning. These programs succeed to a degree. However, why do some learners do so well while others do not? In Edu-K we see that some individuals try too hard and "switch off" the brain-integration mechanisms necessary for complete learning. Information is received by the back brain as an "impress" but is inaccessible to the front brain as an "express." This inability to express what is learned locks the student into a failure syndrome.

The solution is whole-brain learning, through movement repatterning and through Brain Gym activities that enable students to access those parts of the brain previously inaccessible to them. The changes in learning and behavior are often immediate and profound, as children discover how to receive information and express themselves simultaneously.

Other books in this series include *Edu-K for Kids*, which teaches the repatterning procedures recommended for everyone who wants to improve the quality of his or her living, learning, and enjoyment of movement. The *Brain Gym* book teaches simple activities which have changed many lives since they were first introduced. Although Brain Gym activities will help any individual, young or old, to make better use of innate learning potential, they are most effective after Dennison Laterality Repatterning (described in *Edu-K for Kids*). This teacher's edition offers a more in-depth explanation of the Brain Gym movements and whole-brain learning concepts.

For more than fifty years, pioneers in behavioral optometry and sensorimotor training have provided statistical research showing the effects of movement upon learning. Dr. Dennison's familiarity with this research, oriented mainly toward children with specific language disabilities, led him to extrapolate this information into quick, simple, task-specific movements that benefit every learner. These movements of body and energy are appropriate to the special needs of people learning in our modern, highly technological culture. This book was written so that people can experience the vitalizing effects of these movements in their daily-life activities.

Many teachers use all of the Brain Gym movements in their classrooms every day. Others use only the movements related to reading, during the reading hour. Of course, no one should ever be required to move in a way which feels unnatural or uncomfortable. Each student should work within his or her own abilities, and be encouraged, yet never forced, to do any of these activities. People tell us they do these movements automatically, just "knowing" when they can benefit from Brain Gym!

For parents or teachers using the *Brain Gym Teacher's Edition*, the categories entitled ACTIVATES THE BRAIN FOR, ACADEMIC SKILLS, and BEHAVIORAL/POSTURAL CORRELATES may be especially helpful. Often, doing Brain Gym movements for a specific skill will allow the student to make an immediate improvement in behavior or performance. However, in most cases the information will help the parent or teacher guide the learner gradually to long-term benefits.

When students are introduced to Brain Gym, they seem to love it, request it, teach it to their friends, and integrate it into their lives, without any coaching or supervision. The skilled teacher who enjoys movement will inspire that motivation without effort!

Introduction

The *Brain Gym Teacher's Edition* is a companion guide to the *Brain Gym* book, for the use of parents, educators, and others who are actively working with children or adults, individually or in groups, to help them draw out their full potential as learners. The reader will find this an easy-to-use, self-explanatory reference book whenever Brain Gym is being learned. By turning to any one page in the *Teacher's Edition*, the educator will find information and teaching strategies which will enable him or her to explain, refine, and vary the activity for a particular individual, situation, or need. Included on each page is information under the following headings:

TEACHING TIPS   ACADEMIC SKILLS
VARIATIONS   BEHAVIORAL/POSTURAL CORRELATES
ACTIVATE(S) THE BRAIN FOR RELATED MOVEMENTS
            HISTORY OF THE MOVEMENT

As explained in the histories of the movements, these Brain Gym activities were discovered to either stimulate (Laterality Dimension), release (Focusing Dimension), or relax (Centering Dimension) students involved in particular types of learning situations. Specific activities were observed to be more helpful than others for moving through individual learning blocks, and a pattern was recognized. This *Teacher's Edition* can guide the educator or parent to observe and recognize these patterns and thus make facilitation of the learning experience more precise and accurate.

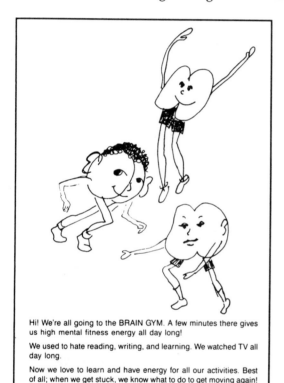

Hi! We're all going to the BRAIN GYM. A few minutes there gives us high mental fitness energy all day long!

We used to hate reading, writing, and learning. We watched TV all day long.

Now we love to learn and have energy for all our activities. Best of all; when we get stuck, we know what to do to get moving again!

The human brain, like a hologram, is three-dimensional, with parts interrelating as a whole. Thus, the infant or preschool child is capable of globally taking in the adult world and recreating it; the student easily integrates learning presented from a multisensory, rather than abstract, orientation. However, the human brain is also task-specific, and, for the purposes of applying Brain Gym movements, may be understood to comprise the left and right hemispheres (Laterality Dimension), the brainstem and frontal lobes (Focus Dimension), and the limbic system and cerebral cortex (Centering Dimension).

Within laterality, or sidedness, exists the potential for bilateral integration, the ability to cross the central midline of the body and to work in the midfield. When this skill is mastered, one can process a linear, symbolic, written code, left to right or right to left, an ability fundamental to academic success (see *Edu-K for Kids*). The inability to cross the midline results in such identifications as "learning disabled" or "dyslexic." Those movements which will help to stimulate bihemispheric and bilateral integration are so identified under the ACTIVATE(S) THE BRAIN FOR category.

Focusing is the ability to cross the participation midline, which separates the back and front of the body as well as the back (occipital) and frontal lobes. Incompletion of developmental reflexes results in the inability to express oneself with ease and to participate actively in the learning process. Students who are underfocused are often labelled as "inattentive," "unable to comprehend," "language-delayed," or "hyperactive." Some children are overfocused and try too hard. Those movements which help to unblock focus are designated as back/front integration activities under the ACTIVATE(S) THE BRAIN FOR category.

Centering is the ability to cross the midline between the upper and lower body and the corresponding upper and lower brain functions: the midbrain (emotional content) and cerebrum (abstract thought). Nothing can be truly learned without feeling and a sense of meaningfulness. The inability to stay centered results in irrational fear, fight-or-flight responses, or an inability to feel or express emotions. Those movements which relax the system and prepare the student to take in and process information without negative emotional overlay are identified by the centering or grounding designation under the ACTIVATE(S) THE BRAIN FOR category.

Once the student learns to move his or her eyes, hands, and body in concert, the Brain Gym activities have served their purpose, and integration becomes an automatic choice. Some individuals will find Brain Gym helpful over a short period of time to establish a desired behavior. Most students consciously choose to continue the movements for a matter of weeks or months, to help reinforce the new learning. Many learners will return to their favorite Brain Gym movement routine when new stresses or challenges appear in their lives.

Brain Gym is based upon three simple premises:
1. Learning is a natural, joyous activity that continues throughout life.
2. Learning blocks are the inability to move through the stress and uncertainty of a new task.
3. We are all "learning-blocked" to the extent that we have learned not to move.

Many of us have come to accept limitations in our lives as inevitable, and may fail to find the benefits that positive stress can bring. The Brain Gym movements are a natural, healthful alternative to tension that we can use and teach others to use when challenges present themselves.

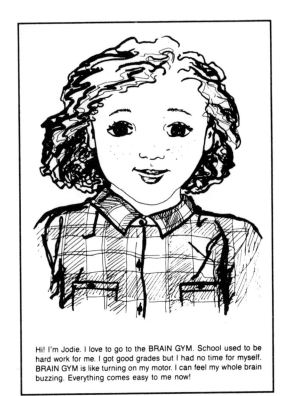

The educator, in particular, must be an expert at identifying behaviors that indicate that the student is having difficulty moving information through to integration. With Brain Gym, most learning blocks can be released if they are recognized and addressed in a supportive manner.

The healthy child knows when he or she is stuck, and asks for help by means of his or her behavior. There are no lazy, withdrawn, aggressive, or angry children, only children denied the ability to learn in a way that is natural to them.

Hi! I'm Jodie. I love to go to the BRAIN GYM. School used to be hard work for me. I got good grades but I had no time for myself. BRAIN GYM is like turning on my motor. I can feel my whole brain buzzing. Everything comes easy to me now!

Given the opportunity to move in his own way, the child is capable of completing the learning cycle. With support, and with permission to move in the classroom in a positive manner, he will unfold into his unique and complete intelligence in a way that is natural and easy. He will not be blocked; he will be free to learn.

The Midline Movements

The Midline Movements focus on the skills necessary for easy two-sided (left-right) movement across the midline of the body. The vertical midline of the body is the necessary reference for all such bilateral skills. The midfield (first defined by Dr. Dennison) is the area where the left and right visual fields overlap, requiring the paired eyes and all of their reciprocating muscles to work so well as a team that the two eyes function as one. Development of bilateral movement skills for crawling, walking, or seeing depth is essential to the child's growing sense of autonomy. It is also a prerequisite for whole-body coordination and ease of learning in the near-visual area. The Midline Movements help to integrate binocular vision, binaural hearing, and the left and right sides of the brain and body.

Many learners beginning school are not developmentally prepared for the bilateral, two-dimensional skills of near-point work. Sometimes a student is coordinated for play or sports activities (involving three-dimensional space and demanding binocular vision only beyond arm's length), yet is not ready to use both eyes, ears, hands, and brain hemispheres for near-point work, such as reading, writing, and other skills involving fine-motor coordination. Other students show coordination for academic skills or near-point activities, yet are not ready for whole-body coordination on the playing field. The Midline Movements facilitate completion of developmental skills and give the learner permission to build on the concrete operations already established. They help students to increase upper-lower body coordination, for both large-motor activities and fine-motor skills.

Cross-motor activities have been used to activate the brain since our understanding of laterality began over a century ago. Noted authorities such as Orton, Doman, Delacato, Kephart, and Barsch have used similar movements successfully in their learning programs. Dr. Dennison drew from his knowledge of these programs in developing the Midline Movements series.

Paul Dennison has worked closely with behavioral optometrists for more than twenty years. He recognizes the value of perceptual-motor and vision training for certain students, and has included his own movement innovations for releasing visual stress and creating eye-teaming skills.

Some of the Midline Movements have been adapted from activities used in behavioral optometry to increase brain-body coordination. Others are borrowed from sports, dance, or exercise programs. Still others, totally unique to Edu-K, are the innovations of Dr. Paul Dennison.

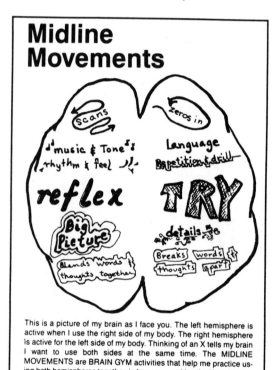

Midline Movements

This is a picture of my brain as I face you. The left hemisphere is active when I use the right side of my body. The right hemisphere is active for the left side of my body. Thinking of an X tells my brain I want to use both sides at the same time. The MIDLINE MOVEMENTS are BRAIN GYM activities that help me practice using both hemispheres together, in harmony, making the X work better and better!

CROSS CRAWL

In this contralateral exercise, similar to walking in place, the student alternately moves one arm and its opposite leg and the other arm and *its* opposite leg. Because Cross Crawl accesses both brain hemispheres simultaneously, this is the ideal warm-up for all skills which require crossing the body's lateral midline.

TEACHING TIPS

- Water and Brain Buttons help prepare the body and brain to respond to Cross Crawl.
- To activate the kinesthetic sense, alternately touch each hand to the opposite knee.

VARIATIONS

- Cross Crawl as you sit, moving opposite arm and leg together.
- Reach with opposite arm and leg in varied directions.
- Reach behind the body to touch the opposite foot. (See *Switching On* for more variations.)
- Do a slow-motion Cross Crawl, reaching opposite arm and leg to their full extension (Cross Crawl for focus).
- Skip (or bounce lightly) between each Cross Crawl. (Skip-Across is especially helpful for centering; it also alleviates visual stress.)
- To improve balance, Cross Crawl with your eyes closed, or pretend to swim while Cross Crawling.
- Use color-coded stickers or ribbons on opposite hands and feet for children who may need this clue.
- Do Cross Crawl to a variety of music and rhythms.

ACTIVATES THE BRAIN FOR

- crossing the visual/auditory/kinesthetic/tactile midline
- left-to-right eye movements
- improved binocular (both eyes together) vision

ACADEMIC SKILLS

- spelling
- writing
- listening
- reading and comprehension

BEHAVIORAL/POSTURAL CORRELATES

- improved left/right coordination
- enhanced breathing and stamina
- greater coordination and spatial awareness
- enhanced hearing and vision

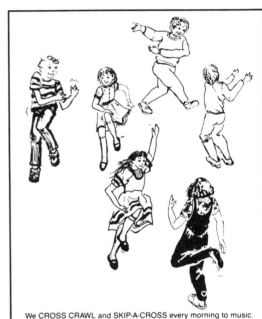

We CROSS CRAWL and SKIP-A-CROSS every morning to music. I coordinate the movement so that when an arm moves, the leg on the opposite side of the body moves at the same time. I move to the front, sides, and back and move my eyes in all directions. It helps to touch my hand to the opposite knee occasionally to "cross the midline". When my brain hemispheres work together like this, I really feel open to learning new things.

RELATED MOVEMENTS

Lazy 8s, p. 5
Brain Buttons, p. 25
The Thinking Cap, p. 30

HISTORY OF THE MOVEMENT

As the body grows, interweaving of the opposite sides through movement naturally occurs during such activities as crawling, walking, and running. Over the last century, crawling has been used in neurological patterning to maximize learning potential. Experts theorized that contralateral movements worked by activating the speech and language centers of the brain. However, Dr. Dennison discovered that Cross Crawl activity is effective because it stimulates the receptive as well as expressive hemisphere of the brain, faciliting integrated learning. This preference for whole-brain movement over one-side-at-a-time processing can be established through Dennison Laterality Repatterning (see *Edu-K for Kids*).

LAZY 8s

Drawing the Lazy 8 or infinity symbol enables the reader to cross the visual midline without interruption, thus activating both right and left eyes and integrating the right and left visual fields. The 8 is drawn on its side and includes a definite midpoint and separate left and right areas, joined by a continuous line.

TEACHING TIPS

- The student aligns his body with a point at eye level. This will be the midpoint of the 8.
- The student chooses a comfortable position for drawing the Lazy 8, adjusting the width and height to fit his needs. (It's best to involve one's full visual field and the full extension of both arms.)
- The student may use the left hand first, to activate the right hemisphere immediately.
- He starts on the midline and moves counterclockwise first: up, over, and around. Then from his waist he moves clockwise: up, over, around, and back to the beginning midpoint.
- As the eyes follow the Lazy 8, the head moves slightly and the neck remains relaxed.
- Three repetitions with each hand separately, then with both together, are recommended. Two colors of chalk or ink may be used.

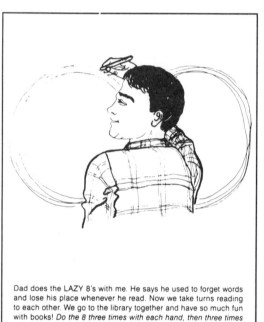

Dad does the LAZY 8's with me. He says he used to forget words and lose his place whenever he read. Now we take turns reading to each other. We go to the library together and have so much fun with books! Do the 8 three times with each hand, then three times with both hands together.

VARIATIONS

- Involve auditory processing and teach left and right by saying, "Up to the left and around. Cross the middle and up. Around, down, and back to the middle."
- The student may do the movement with eyes closed to increase his kinesthetic sense of the Lazy 8.
- Humming while doing the Lazy 8 may increase relaxation.
- Draw the Lazy 8 in the air, with streamers, or against different tactile surfaces, like sand, the paper, or chalkboard.
- Graduate the 8 from larger to smaller sizes, drawn first on a large surface parallel to the face, and later at a desk, so the movement is connected to writing.
- Energy 8's: Swing both arms simultaneously down, across each other, then up and over. Move arms slowly, being aware of both left and right visual fields, and quickly, soft-focusing on the afterimage of the arms.

ACTIVATE THE BRAIN FOR

- crossing the visual midline for increased hemispheric integration
- enhanced binocular and peripheral vision
- improved eye-muscle coordination (especially for tracking)

ACADEMIC SKILLS

- the mechanics of reading (left-to-right eye movement)
- symbol recognition for the decoding of written language
- reading comprehension (long-term associative memory)

BEHAVIORAL/POSTURAL CORRELATES

- relaxation of eyes, neck, and shoulders while focusing
- improved depth perception
- improved centering, balance, and coordination

RELATED MOVEMENTS

Brain Buttons, p. 25
Cross Crawl, p. 4
Double Doodle, p. 6

HISTORY OF THE MOVEMENT

Tracing or feeling movement along a small infinity sign or "Lazy 8" has been used in educational therapy to develop kinesthetic and tactile awareness in students with severe learning problems. These students are not yet ready neurologically to cross the visual midline. The movement results in the elimination of reversals and transpositions in reading and writing. Dr. Dennison adapted the Lazy 8 as part of his vision-training work in 1974 by having students use their large muscles to draw Lazy 8s on the chalkboard, the eyes following the hand movement. His students showed immediate improvement in the ability to discriminate symbols and to know their left from their right sides.

DOUBLE DOODLE

Double Doodle is a bilateral drawing activity which is done in the midfield to establish direction and orientation in space relative to the body. When the learner has developed a sense of left-and-right discrimination, as she draws and writes she experiences herself in the center, and movement toward, away from, up, and down is interpreted in relationship to that center. Prior to developing this sense, the child fumbles to recreate a shape from memory.

The Double Doodle is best experienced with the large muscles of the arms and shoulders. Stand behind the student and guide her arms and hands through a few simple movements. Teach the student to refer to her physical midline for directional reference. Say "Out, up, in, and down" as you guide the student to draw squares with both hands simultaneously. Set the student free when both hands are able to move together, mirroring each other easily.

TEACHING TIPS
- Begin by allowing the student to freeform "scribble" with both hands together (as in fingerpainting).
- The student starts with large arm movements, neck and eyes relaxed, working at a large board.
- Emphasize the process, not the product. Avoid making either positive or negative judgments.
- Encourage relaxed head and eye movements.
- Have samples of Double Doodle shapes that others have done.
- Encourage innovation and experimentation.
- Double Doodling of actual shapes, like circles, triangles, stars, hearts, trees, or faces, is most fun when done spontaneously.

VARIATIONS
- Progress from the large board to a smaller piece of paper taped to the desk or floor.
- Offer different tools for doing Double Doodle (e.g., chalk, paint, markers, crayons.)
- Double Doodle in the air as a group activity.
- Double Doodle touching different fingers to the thumbs (releasing thumb/index finger tensions).
- Doodle in the air with shoulders, elbows, wrists, or feet (relaxes tensions).
- Quadroodle Doodle: Doodle with hands and feet at the same time.

ACTIVATES THE BRAIN FOR
- hand-eye coordination in different visual fields
- crossing the kinesthetic midline
- spatial awareness and visual discrimination

ACADEMIC SKILLS
- following directions
- decoding and encoding of written symbols
- writing; spelling; math

BEHAVIORAL/POSTURAL CORRELATES
- left and right awareness
- improved peripheral vision
- body awareness, coordination, and specialization of hands and eyes
- improved sports abilities and movement skills

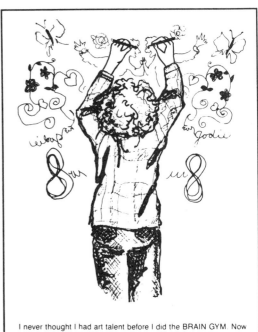

I never thought I had art talent before I did the BRAIN GYM. Now I do the DOUBLE DOODLE, drawing with both hands at the same time, "in," "out," "up," and "down!" I'm always surprised by the interesting shapes I create, and at how relaxed my arms and eyes feel. Writing is much easier for me now, too.

RELATED MOVEMENTS
Lazy 8s, p. 5   Alphabet 8s, p. 7   The Elephant, p. 8

HISTORY OF THE MOVEMENT

Dr. Gettman, an optometrist specializing in developmental vision, described bilateral drawing in his first book, *How to Improve Your Child's Intelligence*. Dr. Dennison adapted this activity for his learning-center students, encouraging creativity, play, and innovation. Double Doodle helps develop eye-teaming skills, eye-hand coordination, handedness, visual convergence, and use of the midfield. When vision improves, academic performance often shows a parallel improvement.

ALPHABET 8s

Alphabet 8s adapt the Lazy 8 form to the printing of lower-case letters from *a* through *t* (these letters evolved from the Arabic system; letters *u* through *z* come from the Roman alphabet). This activity integrates the movements involved in the formation of these letters, enabling the writer to cross the visual midline without confusion. Each letter is clearly superimposed on either one side or the other (see illustration). A downstroke either ends the letter or begins another letter. For most students, when the printing of the lower-case letters improves, handwriting also becomes easier.

TEACHING TIPS

- The student does Lazy 8s (see page 5) before beginning this activity.
- This activity is performed on a large scale first, drawn on the board or in the air with hands clasped together, to activate the large muscles in the arms, shoulders, and chest.
- Note that letters in the left visual field begin on the midline and move "up, around, and down."
- Note that letters in the right visual field begin on the midline or move "down, up, and around."
- Help students discover the structural similarities between letters (e.g., "see the *r* in the *m* and the *n*").

VARIATIONS

- Face student to teach the Alphabet 8s. Clasp her hands in yours, bend your knees, and move with the description and rhythm of each letter (you trace the mirror image).

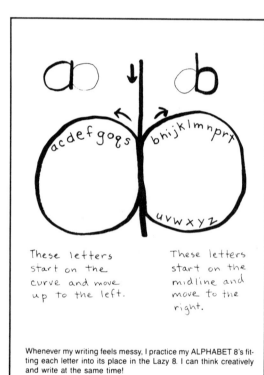

These letters start on the curve and move up to the left.

These letters start on the midline and move to the right.

Whenever my writing feels messy, I practice my ALPHABET 8's fitting each letter into its place in the Lazy 8. I can think creatively and write at the same time!

- Involve auditory/visual/kinesthetic/tactile integration by saying for each letter, "up, around, and down" or "down, up, and around."
- Trace the letters in sand or against different tactile surfaces to feel the flow.
- Do the movement with eyes closed; add humming.
- Alphabet 8s may be done smaller (in handwriting size), when sufficient practice and integration of the large muscles has been experienced.
- Write the letters of spelling words in the Alphabet 8 form.

ACTIVATE THE BRAIN FOR

- crossing the kinesthetic/tactile midline for bihemispheric writing on the midfield
- increased peripheral awareness
- eye-hand coordination
- symbol recognition and discrimination

ACADEMIC SKILLS

- fine-motor skills
- penmanship
- cursive writing
- spelling
- creative writing

BEHAVIORAL/POSTURAL CORRELATES

- relaxation of eyes, neck, shoulders, and wrists while writing
- improved concentration while writing
- greater skill in activities involving eye-hand coordination

RELATED MOVEMENTS

Arm Activation, p. 18   Neck Rolls, p. 9   Double Doodle, p. 6

HISTORY OF THE MOVEMENT

The figure 8 has been used for many years in Special Education and perception training to help students with severe "dyslexia" and "dysgraphia." Dr. Dennison was introduced to figure 8s for writing in 1974 as part of an in-service program at his learning centers in California, and immediately began including them, in a larger size, in his own program, to develop eye-hand coordination and other visual skills. Repatterning students for the alphabet via the Alphabet 8s is one of Dr. Dennison's unique adaptations of the movement.

THE ELEPHANT

The grace and balance for which elephants are known inspired this movement. A bull elephant of the Indian species might weigh over 9,000 pounds, yet every square centimeter of its large foot pad carries only twenty-one pounds of weight (a one hundred twenty-pound woman, by comparison, might exert as much as four and one-half pounds on every square centimeter of her high-heeled shoes). The ears of the East African elephant account for one-third of his total body-surface area. His auditory ability may account in part for his well-developed intelligence.

The Elephant movement activates the inner ear for improved balance and equilibrium and also integrates the brain for listening with both ears. It releases tight neck muscles, which often tense in reaction to sound or to excessive lip movement during silent reading. In the Elephant movement, the torso, head, and pointing arm and hand function as a single unit. This unit moves around a distant, imaginary Lazy 8, eyes focusing beyond the hand. The whole body moves without any separate arm movements.

TEACHING TIPS
- Show the student where to paint the 8 before beginning. Relate the center and sides of the 8 to a shape in the environment (e.g., the center line of the chalkboard).
- The student stands with knees comfortably bent, facing the center of the Lazy 8.
- Pre- and post-test the student's ease of head-turning before and after the movement.
- While keeping both eyes open, the student projects the 8 onto a distant lateral plane with the center of the Lazy 8 at his midline. No body twist is involved.
- The head is "glued" to the shoulder (holding a paper between the head and the shoulder helps with this skill).
- The student aims with his hand, looking past the hand into the distance (the hand will appear double or out of focus if both eyes are correctly processing information).

VARIATIONS
- The student may do the Elephant while sitting.
- The student may point his arm into different visual fields, relaxing different areas of tension.

ACTIVATES THE BRAIN FOR
- crossing the auditory midline (including skills of attention, recognition, perception, discrimination, and memory)
- listening to one's own speaking voice
- short- and long-term memory
- silent speech and thinking ability
- integrating vision, listening, and whole-body movement
- depth perception and eye-teaming ability

ACADEMIC SKILLS
- listening comprehension
- speech
- spelling (decoding: hearing separate syllables and words; encoding: blending syllables together to make words, or blending words to make whole thoughts)
- memory for sequences, as in math or digit spans

BEHAVIORAL/POSTURAL CORRELATES
- left and right head-turning ability
- binocular vision
- a relaxed neck while focusing
- the coordination of upper body and lower body
- activates the inner ear for a sense of balance; especially helpful for jet lag or motion sickness

Mom and I do the ELEPHANT together. She says it relaxes her neck and eyes. I like to write my spelling words (and times tables) in the air with my "trunk". This way I never forget them! The ELEPHANT helps me be a better listener, too. *Bend your knees, "glue" your head to your shoulder, and point across the room. Use your ribs to move your whole upper body as you trace a Lazy 8. Look past your fingers (if you see two hands, that's okay!) Repeat with the other arm.*

RELATED MOVEMENTS
The Thinking Cap, p. 30
The Owl, p. 17

HISTORY OF THE MOVEMENT
Paul E. Dennison, Ph.D., created the Edu-K Elephant in 1981. His insight to adapt the Lazy 8 to stimulate listening and silent-speech skills came out of his knowledge of the development of thinking skills and of their relationship to involuntary movement of the neck muscles, as detected by biofeedback procedures.

NECK ROLLS

Neck Rolls relax the neck and release tensions resulting from an inability to cross the visual midline or to work in the midfield. When done before reading and writing, they encourage binocular vision and binaural hearing. Roll the head in the forward position only. Complete rotations to the back are not recommended.

TEACHING TIPS

- The student allows her head to roll slowly from side to side, as though it were a heavy ball, as she breathes deeply.
- As the head moves, the chin in its extreme positions does not pass either end of the clavicle.
- Be aware of tight spots or tension, and hold the head in that position, breathing deeply, until the neck releases.
- As you move the head, imagine it reaching out of the body, rather than collapsing down.
- Do neck rolls with eyes closed, then with eyes open.

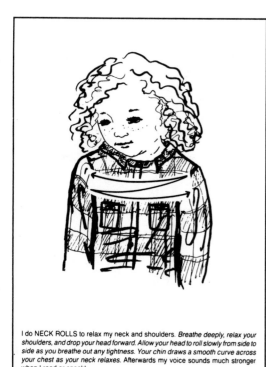

I do NECK ROLLS to relax my neck and shoulders. *Breathe deeply, relax your shoulders, and drop your head forward. Allow your head to roll slowly from side to side as you breathe out any tightness. Your chin draws a smooth curve across your chest as your neck relaxes.* Afterwards my voice sounds much stronger when I read or speak!

VARIATIONS

- Begin with eyes closed. Take several deep, complete breaths. Imagine that your head is a beautiful sculpture resting in perfect balance on a polished post. Move your head in small circles, letting it find its ideal balance point.
- Move the head into a position of tension and do tiny circles with your chin. To further relax tensions, do Lazy 8s or tiny rolls from side to side. Keep moving out in ever larger circles or 8s.
- With one hand, press gently against any point of tension in the base of the head while tracing small circles or Lazy 8s with your nose.
- To improve mouth position and alignment of the jaw where there are speech or tongue-thrust difficulties, rest the teeth together lightly and flatten the tongue like a blanket against the upper palate while doing the movement.
- Complete the Neck Rolls by imagining a warm waterfall flowing down the back of your neck.

ACTIVATE THE BRAIN FOR

- binocular vision and the ability to read and write in the midfield
- centering
- grounding
- relaxation of the central nervous system

ACADEMIC SKILLS

- oral reading
- silent reading, study skills
- speech and language

BEHAVIORAL/POSTURAL CORRELATES

- improved breathing
- increased relaxation

RELATED MOVEMENTS

The Owl, p. 17
The Energizer, p. 14
Brain Buttons, p. 25

HISTORY OF THE MOVEMENT

At times of fatigue, people automatically use neck rolls to vitalize the brain. Dr. Dennison discovered that students who could not cross the midline when reading were often immediately able to do so after a session of neck rolls. This movement is a natural part of kinesthetic learning in which the infant, resting on forearms in a prone posture, gradually develops balanced positions of the jaw, tongue, and neck.

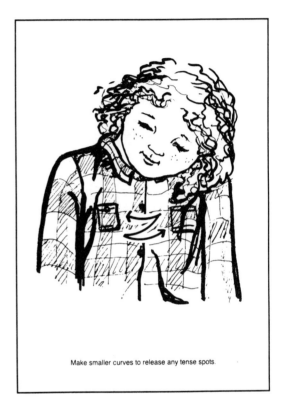

Make smaller curves to release any tense spots.

THE ROCKER

The Rocker releases the low back and sacrum by massaging the hamstring and gluteus muscle groups, stimulating nerves in the hips dulled by excessive sitting (e.g., at desks or in motor vehicles). When the sacrum is freed to move, the brain, at the other end of the central nervous system, is activated as well. Circulation of cerebrospinal fluid within the spinal column is then stimulated, and the body works more efficiently.

TEACHING TIPS

- In order to protect the tailbone, the student does the Rocker on a padded surface.
- Guide the student to use his hands or forearms for support.
- Encourage the student to release tension in first one hip, then the other, by rocking in small circles.

VARIATIONS

- In a chair, the student holds the sides of the chair seat to support himself as he lifts his feet and rocks.
- Students may work in pairs: one person sits alongside the other and places his arms around her knees and back to support them while moving her body in small circles to massage the hip area.

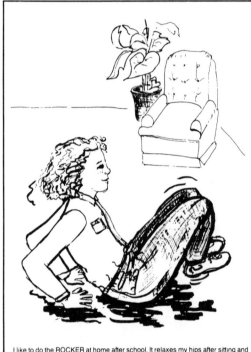

I like to do the ROCKER at home after school. It relaxes my hips after sitting and taking notes. I lean back onto my hands and massage my hips and the back of my legs, rocking myself in circles, back and forth, until the tension melts. Always do the ROCKER on a comfortable surface, like a padded mat.

ACTIVATES THE BRAIN FOR

- centering and the ability to work in the midfield
- study skills
- left-to-right visual skills
- skills of attention and comprehension

RELATED SKILLS

- operating machines: computers, motor vehicles

BEHAVIORAL/POSTURAL CORRELATES

- increased focus and more forward body posture
- the ability to sit squarely in a chair
- a stable pelvis (relaxes swayback, releases torque in hips)
- a less overfocused posture
- knees not locked; hips, shoulders, eyes more level
- deeper breathing and more voice resonance
- increased whole-body coordination
- an increased energy level (alleviates mental fatigue)

RELATED MOVEMENTS

Cross Crawl, p. 4

Belly Breathing, p. 12

The Energizer, p. 14

The Gravity Glider, p. 21

HISTORY OF THE MOVEMENT

At about eight months of age, when a balanced sitting posture is being developed, the infant establishes body rotation toward the midline and coordination between the occiput and sacrum. This important relationship of the sacrum to the base of the skull has been noticed and researched by osteopaths and doctors of chiropractic (especially those practicing the Sacro-Occipital Technique, known as SOT). Dr. Dennison discovered that students who were unable to focus on and comprehend the material they were reading would often be able to do so after doing the Rocker.

BELLY BREATHING

Belly Breathing reminds the student to breathe instead of holding his breath during focused mental activity or physical exertion. The breath should expand the rib cage front to back, left to right, and top to bottom, including the abdomen. When breathing is shallow, lifting only the rib cage, the oxygen supply to the brain is limited. When one breathes correctly, there is abundant oxygen for higher brain functions.

TEACHING TIPS

- The student inhales through the nose and initially cleanses the lungs with one long exhalation, released in short puffs through pursed lips (he may imagine keeping a feather afloat). Thereafter, the outbreath is also through the nose.
- The hand rests on the lower abdomen, rising on inhalation and falling on exhalation.
- Inhale to a count of three, hold breath for three, exhale for three, hold for three. Repeat. For an alternate rhythm, inhale for two, exhale for four, with no holding.
- Ideally, rhythmic breathing is automatic. Rhythmic music may help, so that counting isn't needed.
- When doing activities like lifting, kicking, or pushing, remember to exhale on the exertion.

VARIATIONS

- Lie flat with a book on the belly. The abdomen should rise on inhalation and lower on exhalation.
- 3-D Breathing 8s: Squat with hands flat on the floor, between your knees, to experience the diaphragm as you breathe. Then paint an imaginary 8 between your left and right ribs, feeling both spheres of the 8 expand as you inhale and contract as you exhale. Now turn the 8 so that it expands between your stomach and spine; now turn it top to bottom, expanding your chest and lower abdomen. Can you activate all three 8s at once?
- Paint an 8 on any of the above-mentioned body planes. Let your breath move you as you inhale, painting one side, and exhale, painting the other. Direct the 8 around areas of tension, or around the focal points of any other Brain Gym movement (e.g., your two hands, while you are doing Brain Buttons).
- Walk and Belly Breathe at the same time.

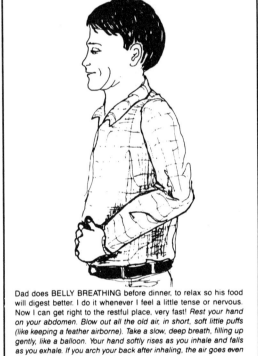

Dad does BELLY BREATHING before dinner, to relax so his food will digest better. I do it whenever I feel a little tense or nervous. Now I can get right to the restful place, very fast! *Rest your hand on your abdomen. Blow out all the old air, in short, soft little puffs (like keeping a feather airborne). Take a slow, deep breath, filling up gently, like a balloon. Your hand softly rises as you inhale and falls as you exhale. If you arch your back after inhaling, the air goes even deeper.*

ACTIVATES THE BRAIN FOR

- the ability to cross the midline
- centering and grounding
- relaxation of the central nervous system
- cranial rhythms

ACADEMIC SKILLS

- reading (encoding and decoding)
- speech and oral reading

BEHAVIORAL/POSTURAL CORRELATES

- improved inflection and expression
- a heightened energy level
- diaphragmatic breathing
- an improved attention span

RELATED MOVEMENTS

The Rocker, p. 11
The Energy Yawn, p. 29
See also: Lengthening Activities, pp. 17-22

HISTORY OF THE MOVEMENT

Breathing is ideally an automatic ability that adjusts itself to fit the task. Some people have incorrectly learned to hold their breath as part of the tendon-guard reflex (see Lengthening Activities, p. 16). Often students who have learned to breathe properly for singing or playing an instrument show the advantage in their reading skills. For some, though, self-conscious attempts to control the breath only add to the stress around breathing. Dr. Dennison has taught Belly Breathing to his reading students after the tendon-guard reflex has been released, with excellent results. Blocked, labored breathing becomes natural and spontaneous, and there is more oxygen, and thus energy, available for thinking, speaking, and moving.

CROSS CRAWL SIT-UPS

Cross Crawl Sit-ups strengthen the abdominals, relax the lower back, and activate the integration of the left and right brain hemispheres. They develop coordination of the core, postural muscles and a sense of organization around the body's midline.

TEACHING TIPS

- The student does Cross Crawl Sit-ups on a padded surface to protect the tailbone.
- The student does the movement while positioned on his back. The knees and head are up, and the hands are clasped behind the head for support.
- The student touches one elbow to the opposite knee, then alternates his movement as though riding a bicycle; his neck stays relaxed and breathing is rhythmic.
- The student imagines an X connecting his hips and shoulders, increasing awareness of his abdominals.

VARIATIONS

- The student lies flat, with arms overhead and legs extended. He lifts one knee and touches it with the opposite hand, as in standing Cross Crawl. This strengthens the abdominal muscles for students who are uncomfortable lifting the head.

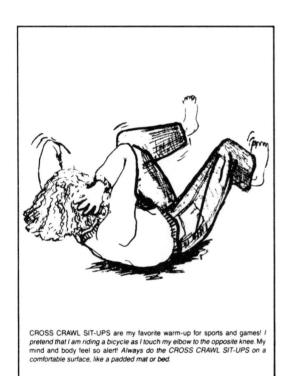

CROSS CRAWL SIT-UPS are my favorite warm-up for sports and games! I pretend that I am riding a bicycle as I touch my elbow to the opposite knee. My mind and body feel so alert! Always do the CROSS CRAWL SIT-UPS on a comfortable surface, like a padded mat or bed.

ACTIVATE THE BRAIN FOR

- left-right integration
- centering and grounding
- awareness of core, postural muscles

ACADEMIC SKILLS

- reading (decoding and encoding)
- listening skills
- math (computations)
- the mechanics of spelling and writing

BEHAVIORAL/POSTURAL CORRELATES

- strengthened abdominal muscles
- a relaxed, strong lumbar spine (lower back)
- diaphragm moves separately from stomach muscles

RELATED MOVEMENTS

Cross Crawl, p. 4

Lazy 8s, p. 5

Brain Buttons, p. 25

The Thinking Cap, p. 30

HISTORY OF THE MOVEMENT

Traditional sit-ups can create strain or imbalance in back and leg muscles. People tend to hold their breath and perform sit-ups incorrectly, or else avoid doing them altogether. Cross Crawl Sit-ups are a safe way to strengthen abdominal muscles for optimal functioning. Dr. Dennison discovered that, when he taught this movement, students were better able to coordinate the two sides of the body and brain, and breathing became easier and more automatic. This movement reinforces the tonus of core muscles and the separate control of the head ideally established in the first year of life.

THE ENERGIZER

The student sits comfortably in a chair, head resting on a desk or table. She places her hands on the desk in front of her shoulders, fingers pointing slightly inward. As she inhales she experiences her breath flowing up the midline like a fountain of energy, lifting first her forehead, then her neck, and finally her upper back. Her diaphragm and chest stay open and her shoulders stay relaxed. The release is just as important as the lift; she curls her head toward her chest, then brings her forehead down to rest on the desk. This back-and-forward movement of the head increases circulation to the frontal lobe for greater comprehension and rational thinking.

TEACHING TIPS

- Keep the shoulders apart and relaxed.
- Remember to breathe into the base of the spine.
- Experience your breath (rather than your muscles) as the source of your strength.
- Repeat the movement three times, noting how it is easier with each repetition.

VARIATIONS

- The Energizer can be done face down on a mat. The student relaxes her body, placing her hands under her shoulders with palms against the mat. She then lifts her head, then her upper back, as before. The hips and lower body stay relaxed, touching the mat.

ACTIVATES THE BRAIN FOR

- the ability to cross the midline
- a relaxed central nervous system

ACADEMIC SKILLS

- binocular vision and eye-teaming skills
- listening comprehension
- speech and language skills
- fine-motor control of eye and hand muscles

BEHAVIORAL/POSTURAL CORRELATES

- improved posture
- enhanced concentration and attention
- improved breathing and voice resonance

RELATED MOVEMENTS

The Owl, p. 17   Belly Breathing, p. 12
Brain Buttons, p. 25

HISTORY OF THE MOVEMENT

Variations on the Energizer are used in many movement disciplines to keep the spine supple, flexible, and relaxed. Increasing the spinal column's range of motion improves lines of communication between the central nervous system and the brain. Developmentally, at about three months the infant begins this upward lifting of the head over the visual midfield.

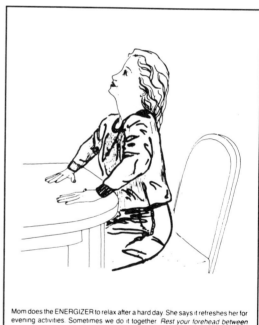

Mom does the ENERGIZER to relax after a hard day. She says it refreshes her for evening activities. Sometimes we do it together. Rest your forehead between your hands. Breathe out all your tension. Then quietly breathe in as the air fills up your midline. Your head easily lifts up, forehead first, followed by your neck and upper body. Your lower body and shoulders stay relaxed. Exhale as you tuck your chin down into your chest. Pull your head forward, lengthening the back of your neck. Relax and breathe deeply.

This movement, called the symmetrical tonic neck reflex in child development literature, helps stimulate the forearms for muscle tonus, establishes control of the head, and activates depth perception, coordinating these for later fine-motor skills. In 1974, Dr. Dennison began using variations on the Energizer at his learning centers to reverse the postural stress of desk and computer work or TV watching, which emphasize overconvergence and forward focusing without opportunities to use the opposing muscles.

THINK OF AN X

The X is the brain-organization pattern for crossing the lateral midline (see *Edu-K for Kids* by Dennison and Dennison). Ideally, through completion in infancy of a series of one-sided and cross-lateral developmental steps, the left hemisphere moves the right side of the body and the right hemisphere moves the left. The whole brain learns through movement to work cooperatively, making both sides available for both receptive and expressive processes. The X is also a reminder of the Lazy 8, activating left and right brain hemispheres for both body movement and relaxation, and activating both eyes for binocular vision.

TEACHING TIPS

- Students may remind themselves to respond to situations in the optimal, whole-brained way by "thinking of an X."
- Xs may be posted on signs for students to look at wherever appropriate. The more often students do Cross Crawl and their other Brain Gym activities, the more effective and automatic a reminder the X will become for them.

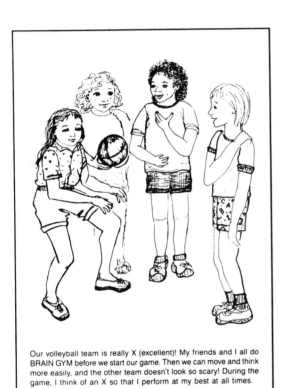

Our volleyball team is really X (excellent)! My friends and I all do BRAIN GYM before we start our game. Then we can move and think more easily, and the other team doesn't look so scary! During the game, I think of an X so that I perform at my best at all times.

VARIATIONS

- Picture the X extending between opposite shoulders and hips, especially during potentially one-sided activities like bicycling, weightlifting, or carrying an object on one side of the body.
- To activate centralized vision, depth perception, and perspective, picture a large X lying flat. The center of the X covers the central point of your focus. Picture the center of the X becoming clearer as the legs of the X fade.

ACTIVATES THE BRAIN FOR

- binocular vision
- binaural hearing
- whole-body coordination
- centralized vision

ACADEMIC SKILLS

- writing
- organization for math or spelling

BEHAVIORAL/POSTURAL CORRELATES

- enhanced concentration and attention
- improved coordination for movement or for sports performance
- enhanced planning or scheduling of priorities

RELATED MOVEMENTS

Cross Crawl, p. 4
Lazy 8s, p. 5
Alphabet 8s, p. 7
Brain Buttons, p. 25

HISTORY OF THE MOVEMENT

Dr. Dennision began using the X in his learning centers to help explain to learners the difference between bilateral, Cross Crawl movements and one-sided movements. Over time, he realized that thinking of the X was a helpful reminder to students to use both visual fields and to coordinate left-right body movements, especially during integration of these skills when they were not completed in the optimal developmental time frame.

Lengthening Activities

The Brain Gym Lengthening Activities help students to develop and reinforce those neural pathways that enable them to make connections between what they already know in the back of the brain and the ability to express and process that information in the front of the brain. These activities are especially effective when used to release reflexes related to specific language disabilities. Learners need to approach the communication skills of reading, writing, listening, and speaking with a sense of adventure, curiosity, and risk-taking. Yet some young people perceive these activities as immediate threats to their survival. The survival mechanism housed in the brainstem is well developed during the first five months of life to take in sensory data from the environment. When placed in new situations where there is too much information, the organism will respond by withdrawing or holding back until there is sufficient comfort to proceed. One physiological reflex to danger is to contract the muscles. This reflex has served over the centuries to protect people from real threats to their lives. It affects posture by shortening the tendons in the back of the body, from head to heels, thus confounding vestibular balance and the sense of spatial relationships.

This contraction response, known as the "tendon-guard reflex" to doctors of chiropractic who practice the Sacro-Occipital Chiropractic Technique (SOT), can become a habit, and is then difficult or impossible to release without training. What is perceived to constitute danger, thus activating the reflex, depends on patterned responses from infancy, and varies for different individuals. Generally, the tendency to contract is lessened as individuals experience a feeling of "participation readiness." The front portion of the brain, especially the frontal lobe, is involved in comprehension, motor control, and rational behaviors necessary for participation in social situations. The Lengthening Activities have been found to relax those muscles and tendons that tighten and shorten by brainstem reflex when we are in unfamiliar learning situations. This resets the proprioceptors, the "brain cells in muscles" that give us information about where we are in space, enabling us to have better access to the whole brain-body system.

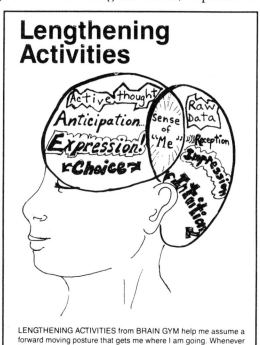

LENGTHENING ACTIVITIES from BRAIN GYM help me assume a forward moving posture that gets me where I am going. Whenever I feel like I'm holding back, or can't express what I know, I do my LENGTHENING ACTIVITIES. Afterwards, I feel more animated, and can enjoy participating again.

The Lengthening Activities may resemble those stretching and limbering exercises done by athletes and dancers in their warm-ups. Although these activities may be used for muscle toning before or after physical exercise, they also serve a different purpose. Each re-educates the body to make lasting changes in posture, restoring muscles to their natural length. Language used to facilitate these movements should describe "reaching, lengthening, expanding," or "opening," rather than "stretching" or "trying," which suggest efforting beyond the natural capacity.

Lengthening Activities also help to develop the sense of participation readiness by releasing or helping to complete infant reflexes that emphasize one-sidedness, crucial to body differentiation and language development. These reflexes continue to demand first priority on neural pathways when individuals have not successfully matured through them. Lengthening Activities address several developmental responses, including the labyrinth responses (birth to four or five months) necessary for development of the inner-ear mechanism and its relationship to gravity; the tonic neck reflexes (birth to three months) critical to the development of sidedness as well as to flexion and erection against gravity; and differentiated movement (birth through childhood), a gradual process of learning to distinguish among the muscles, tendons, and joints of the body, resulting first in gross-motor control and eventually in fine-motor control.

THE OWL

The bird for which this movement is named has a large head, large eyes, and soft feathers that enable him to fly noiselessly. The owl turns his head and eyes at the same time, and has an extremely full range of vision, as he can turn his head over 180 degrees. He also has radar-like hearing. The Owl movement addresses these same visual, auditory, and head-turning skills. It releases neck and shoulder tension that develops under stress, especially when holding a heavy book or when coordinating the eyes for reading or other near-point skills. Further, the Owl releases neck tension caused by subvocalization during reading. It lengthens neck and shoulder muscles, restoring range of motion and circulation of blood to the brain for improved focus, attention, and memory skills.

TEACHING TIPS

- The student squeezes one shoulder to release neck muscles tensed in reaction to listening, speaking, or thinking.
- The student moves his head smoothly across the midfield, to the left, then the right, keeping his chin level.
- The student exhales in each extended head position: to the left and then to the right, and again with the head tilted forward, to release back-of-the-neck muscles. The Owl is repeated with the other shoulder.
- The head may move further into the left and right auditory positions with each release.

VARIATIONS

- While doing the Owl, blink lightly, allowing eye movement to shift along the horizon.
- Add one or two complete breathing cycles in each of the three extended head positions, relaxing fully.
- Emphasize listening with the left ear (head left), right ear (head right), and both ears together (chin down).
- Make a sound (e.g., the owl's "who-o-o") on exhalation.

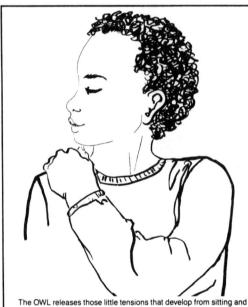

The OWL releases those little tensions that develop from sitting and reading alot. Josh takes a short break to do the OWL, so he will be refreshed for the next lesson. *Grasp the shoulder and squeeze the muscles firmly. Turn your head to look back over your shoulder. Breathe deeply, and pull your shoulders back. Now look over the other shoulder, opening the shoulders again. Drop your chin to your chest, and breathe deeply, letting the muscles relax. Repeat with hand squeezing the opposite shoulder.*

ACTIVATES THE BRAIN FOR

- crossing the "auditory midline" (auditory attention, perception, and memory)
- listening to the sound of one's own voice
- short- and long-term memory
- silent speech and thinking ability
- efficient saccadic eye movement
- integration of vision and listening with whole-body movement

ACADEMIC SKILLS

- listening comprehension
- speech or oral reports
- mathematical computation
- memory (for spelling or digit spans)
- computer or other keyboard work

BEHAVIORAL/POSTURAL CORRELATES

- the ability to turn the head left and right
- strength and balance of front and back neck muscles
- alleviated squinting or staring habits
- relaxed neck, jaw, and shoulder muscles, even when focusing
- head centering (helps release the need to tilt the head or lean on the elbows)
- balanced front- and back-of-the-neck muscles (alleviates overfocused posture)

RELATED MOVEMENTS

The Elephant, p. 8   See also: Arm Activation, p. 18
The Thinking Cap, p. 30

HISTORY OF THE MOVEMENT

The Owl, a self-help release of the upper trapezius muscle, was created by Dr. Dennison as a way to relieve the tension experienced when performing near-point skills such as reading, writing, math calculations, and computer tasks. In the first six months of life, turning the head activates the tonic neck reflex essential to development of both laterality and language. Like the Elephant, this movement re-educates neck-and-shoulder-muscle proprioception related to auditory skills. When this proprioception is re-established, the abilities to listen, think, and access memory are enhanced.

ARM ACTIVATION

Arm Activation is an isometric self-help activity which lengthens the muscles of the upper chest and shoulders. Muscular control for both gross-motor and fine-motor activities originates in this area. If these muscles are shortened from tension, activities related to writing and the control of tools are inhibited.

TEACHING TIPS

- The student experiences her arms as they hang loosely at her sides.
- The student activates one arm as illustrated, while keeping her head relaxed. She then compares the two arms in terms of length, relaxation, and flexibility, before activating the other arm.
- Activation is done in four positions: away from the head, forward, backward, and toward the ear.
- The student may feel the arm activation all the way down to the ribcage.
- The student exhales on the activation, releasing the breath over eight or more counts.
- The student may notice increased relaxation, coordination, and vitality as arm tension is released.
- On completing the movement, the student rolls or shakes her shoulders, noticing the relaxation.

VARIATIONS

- Take more than one complete breath in each position of activation.
- While activating, reach up to further open the diaphragm.
- This can be done sitting, standing, or lying down.
- Arm Activations can be done in different arm positions (e.g., arm straight ahead, next to hip, behind the waist).

ACTIVATES THE BRAIN FOR

- expressive speech and language ability
- relaxed use of diaphragm and increased respiration
- eye-hand coordination and the manipulation of tools

ACADEMIC SKILLS

- penmanship and cursive writing
- spelling
- creative writing

RELATED SKILLS

- operating machines (e.g., a word processor)

BEHAVIORAL/POSTURAL CORRELATES

- an increased attention span for written work
- improved focus and concentration without overfocus
- improved breathing and a relaxed attitude
- an enhanced ability to express ideas
- increased energy in hands and fingers (relaxes writer's cramp)

RELATED MOVEMENTS

The Owl, p. 17   The Rocker, p. 11
Earth Buttons, p. 26   Alphabet 8s, p. 7
Balance Buttons, p. 27

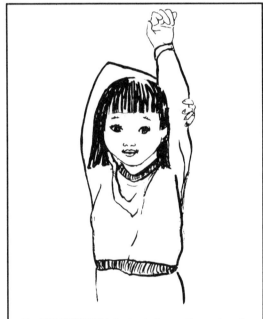

The ARM ACTIVATION helps handwriting, spelling, and creative writing, too! *Hold one arm next to your ear. Exhale gently through pursed lips, while activating the muscles by pushing the arm against the other hand in four directions (front, back, in, and away).* Nikko says her shoulders feel released and she is ready to work.

HISTORY OF THE MOVEMENT

The sense of relationship between moving body parts and a stationary body context (kinesthetic figure-ground) is critical to body stability, especially as distinct movements are developed for eye-hand coordination skills. The toddler gradually begins to differentiate the arms from the body as they are freed from their primary role in balance. Dr. Dennison observed that when gross-motor tensions in the shoulders and chest are released, fine-motor skills are enhanced, facilitating all fine-motor abilities.

THE FOOTFLEX

The Footflex, like the Calf Pump, is a movement re-education process to restore the natural length of the tendons in the feet and lower legs. The tendons shorten to protect the individual from perceived danger, a response caused by a brain reflex to withdraw or to hold back (the tendon-guard reflex). By keeping the calf tendons in the lengthened position while simultaneously activating the foot, the reflex to hold back is relaxed.

TEACHING TIPS

- Sitting with one ankle resting on the other knee, the student places her fingertips at the beginning and end of her calf-muscle area. She might visualize that the tendons and muscles which run from behind the knee to the ankle are like bands of clay. She searches for tight spots at the beginning and end of these bands, and gently holds them apart until they "soften and melt."

- While holding these spots apart, she slowly and methodically points and flexes her foot, extending it farther up and down as this gets easier. The movement is repeated with the other calf and foot.

VARIATIONS

- Find other tense or tender spots along the calf muscles and hold them while pointing and flexing the foot.

- Hold points along the front of the knee and ankle while pointing and flexing the foot, releasing the tibials and the peroneal muscles along the shinbone.

- Straighten the leg in front of you while holding it below the knee and above the ankle, and flex the foot.

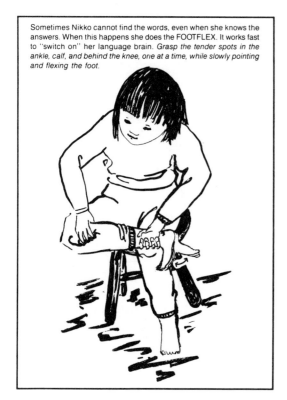

Sometimes Nikko cannot find the words, even when she knows the answers. When this happens she does the FOOTFLEX. It works fast to "switch on" her language brain. *Grasp the tender spots in the ankle, calf, and behind the knee, one at a time, while slowly pointing and flexing the foot.*

ACTIVATES THE BRAIN FOR

- back-front brain integration
- expressive speech and language skills

ACADEMIC SKILLS

- comprehension in listening and reading
- creative writing ability
- the ability to follow through and to complete assignments

BEHAVIORAL/POSTURAL CORRELATES

- a posture that is more forward and relaxed
- knees no longer locked
- improved social behavior
- improved attention span
- increased ability to communicate and respond

RELATED MOVEMENTS

The Calf Pump, p. 20

The Rocker, p. 11

Earth Buttons, p. 26

The Energy Yawn, p. 29

The Grounder, p. 22

Alphabet 8s, p. 7

HISTORY OF THE MOVEMENT

While working with language-delayed children, Dr. Dennison discovered the relationship of the tendons in the calf to self-expression, speech, and language development. Hyperactive children who did not talk were often able to pay attention, listen, learn, and develop language after releasing the calf muscles.

THE CALF PUMP

The Calf Pump, like the Footflex, is a movement re-education process to restore the natural length of the tendons in the feet and lower legs. At times of perceived danger, these tendons shorten to prepare for the act of running (see page 16). By pressing down the heel and lengthening the tendon in the calf, one discharges this fear reflex, and the muscles can return to a normal tonus.

TEACHING TIPS

- The student stands and supports herself with her hands on a wall or on the back of a chair. She places one leg behind her and leans forward, bending the knee of the forward leg. Her straight leg and her back are on one plane.
- In the initial position, the heel at the back is off the floor and the weight is on the forward leg. In the secondary position, weight is shifted to the back leg as the heel is pressed to the floor.
- Exhale while pressing the heel down, releasing with the inhalation. Repeat three or more times.

VARIATIONS

- Further lengthen the tendons by lowering the heel over the edge of a step or block.
- Lengthen the muscles of the upper leg (the hamstrings) by straightening the forward leg and shifting the weight to the back leg.

ACTIVATES THE BRAIN FOR

- back brain-front brain integration
- expressive speech and language ability

ACADEMIC SKILLS

- listening comprehension
- reading comprehension
- creative writing abilities
- the ability to bring processes to closure

BEHAVIORAL/POSTURAL CORRELATES

- improved social behavior
- more prolonged attention span
- an enhanced ability to communicate and respond

RELATED MOVEMENTS

The Footflex, p. 19

The Rocker, p. 11

Earth Buttons, p. 26

The Energy Yawn, p. 29

The Grounder, p. 22

Alphabet 8s, p. 8

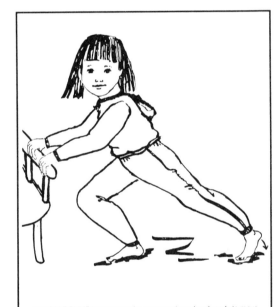

The CALF PUMP helps you to be more motivated and ready to move. We do it whenever we feel "stuck." *As you lean forward and exhale, press the back heel gently to the ground. As you release, lift your heel up and take a deep breath. Repeat three times on each side. The more you bend the forward knee, the more lengthening you feel in the back of the calf.*

HISTORY OF THE MOVEMENT

Dr. Dennison discovered the Calf Pump while working with teens and adults who could not express themselves verbally or write meaningful answers about familiar material. He observed that these individuals locked their knees, activating the tendon-guard reflex and tightening the calf muscles. He modified a hamstring release he had learned as a marathon runner so that it would emphasize the muscles of the calves. The Calf Pump was developed to bring the student's awareness to the calf area, where the instinct to "hold back" originates. Students often become more active participants and are able to access language abilities as soon as the brain reflex to hold back is released.

THE GRAVITY GLIDER

The Gravity Glider is a movement re-education activity to restore the integrity of the hamstrings, hips, and pelvic area. The movement uses balance and gravity to release tension in the hips and pelvis, allowing the student to discover comfortable standing and sitting postures. The student sits comfortably, crossing one foot over the other at the ankles, and reaches forward.

TEACHING TIPS

- The student bends forward, letting gravity take over. He should experience his upper body as fluid, and as separate from the secure base of his legs and hips. Reaching forward from the rib cage allows the legs and the back muscles to lengthen and relax.

- He reaches out in front of him, head down, and allows his arms to glide, extending into all of the places he can reach. His exhalation corresponds to reaching down and forward. Inhalation occurs as he allows his arms and upper body to lift up, parallel to the ground.

- Repeat three times, then change legs.

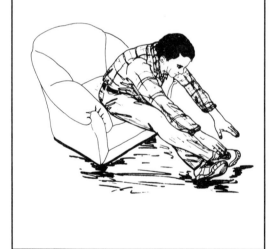

Dad likes to do the GRAVITY GLIDER at work during a long day of sitting at his desk or after driving the car. I do it before my soccer or other sports games. *Sit comfortably. Cross your ankles. Keep your knees relaxed. Bend forward and reach out in front of you, letting your arms glide down as you exhale and up as you inhale. Repeat to the left, right, and center. Change legs and repeat.* My body feels lighter and more relaxed whenever I do this movement.

VARIATIONS

- When ready, do the Gravity Glider with the eyes closed.

- Do the Gravity Glider while standing. Cross the legs at the ankles and establish a comfortable balance. Bending from the hips with the head relaxed down, exhale as you reach slightly out and down with the arms, keeping the knees unlocked and the low back flat.

ACTIVATES THE BRAIN FOR

- a sense of balance and coordination

- a sense of grounding and centering

- increased visual attention (back-front brain integration)

- deeper respiration and increased energy

ACADEMIC SKILLS

- reading comprehension

- mental arithmetic

- abstract thinking in content areas

BEHAVIORAL/POSTURAL CORRELATES

- self-assuredness, confidence, and stability

- self-expression

- the upper and the lower body move as a unified whole

- relaxed posture during extended periods of sitting

RELATED MOVEMENTS

The Calf Pump, p. 20   The Grounder, p. 22
The Footflex, p. 19   The Elephant, p. 8

HISTORY OF THE MOVEMENT

Dr. Dennison learned a standing version of this movement from his modern-dance instructor. After the activity, he was immediately able to move more lightly, and he enjoyed a new sense of balance and of freedom in relation to gravity. Students to whom he taught the Gravity Glider commented on an increased sense of organization within their bodies, and made corresponding academic improvements in organizational skills.

THE GROUNDER

The Grounder is a Lengthening Activity that relaxes the ileopsoas muscle group. These muscles tighten in response to excessive sitting or to stress in the pelvic area, and have the effect of restricting movement and flexibility. This inhibition at the hips locks the sacrum, shortens the breath, and interferes with cranial movement. The ileopsoas muscle group is one of the most important in the body. It is the stabilizing and grounding muscle group for the body, and its flexibility is essential for balance, whole-body coordination, and body focus.

TEACHING TIPS
- The student's feet are positioned about one leg length apart.
- The feet are positioned at right angles to each other.
- The heel of the bent leg is aligned with the instep of the straight leg.
- The bending knee glides, in a straight line, out over the foot, and no farther than the arch.
- The torso and pelvis sit squarely, facing the front; the head, bending knee, and foot of the bent leg face to the side.
- Lengthening occurs in the muscles along the inner hip and thigh of the straight leg.

VARIATIONS
- For a deeper release of the ileopsoas, do the Grounder with the foot of the bent leg on the seat of a chair.
- Lunge forward, the whole body facing the bending leg. Relax in this position, breathing deeply (for limber students only).

ACTIVATES THE BRAIN FOR
- crossing the participation midline
- centering and grounding
- organization
- increased respiration
- spatial awareness
- whole-body relaxation
- relaxed vision

ACADEMIC SKILLS
- comprehension
- long-term recall
- short-term memory storage
- organization for verbal mediation and computation
- self-concept and self-expression

RELATED SKILLS
- keyboard work

BEHAVIORAL/POSTURAL CORRELATES
- greater stability and balance
- improved concentration and attention
- the upper and the lower body move as a unified whole
- hips level (not torqued)
- attitude more grounded and relaxed

HISTORY OF THE MOVEMENT

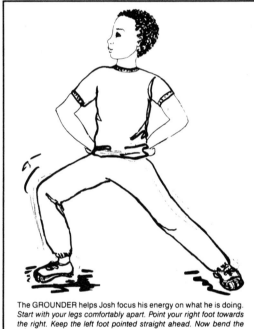

The GROUNDER helps Josh focus his energy on what he is doing. *Start with your legs comfortably apart. Point your right foot towards the right. Keep the left foot pointed straight ahead. Now bend the right knee as you exhale and, then, inhale as you straighten the right leg. Keep your hips tucked under. This strengthens the hip muscles (you feel it in the straight-leg side) and helps stabilize the back. Repeat three times, then repeat on the left side.*

RELATED MOVEMENTS
The Calf Pump, p. 20
The Gravity Glider, p. 21
See also: Belly Breathing, p. 12
Water, p. 24

This gentle lengthening of the ileopsoas muscle was modified by Gail Dennison from a movement posture called "The Archer." Gail recognized the importance of the movement because of her familiarity with Touch for Health and postural integration techniques. The strength and flexibility of the ileopsoas muscle group is also emphasized in dance therapy, sports, and all martial arts. The Grounder safely activates muscle systems that connect, move, and stabilize the upper and lower, left-right, and back-front dimensions of the body. Used in Brain Gym classes since 1984, the Grounder is a valuable addition to the Lengthening Activities.

Energy Exercises and Deepening Attitudes

The Brain Gym Energy Exercises and postures for Deepening Attitudes help to re-establish neural connections between body and brain, thus facilitating the flow of electromagnetic energy throughout the body. These activities support electrical and chemical changes that occur during all mental and physical events. Left-to-right/right-to-left, head-to-foot/foot-to-head, and back-to-front/front-to-back circuitries establish and support our sense of directionality, of sidedness, of centeredness, and of focus, as well as our awareness of where we are in space and in relation to objects in our environment.

The Energy Exercises validate important tactile and kinesthetic information about inner-body relationships that are usually developmentally established during the infant's first year. When visual skills are built on this proprioceptive foundation, a match is easily made between what is seen and what is experienced. Without this congruency, conflict among the sensory channels makes learning difficult.

The human body is one of the most complex of all electrical systems. All visual, auditory, or kinesthetic input–in fact, all sensory information–is changed into electrical signals and relayed to the brain along nerve fibers. The brain then sends out electrical signals along other nerve fibers to tell the visual, auditory, and muscular systems how to respond. These currents travel at speeds of up to 400 kilometers (248 miles) per hour–faster than the fastest electric trains in use!

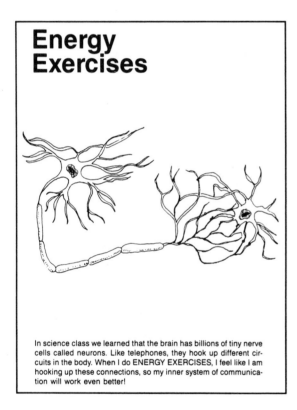

Energy Exercises

In science class we learned that the brain has billions of tiny nerve cells called neurons. Like telephones, they hook up different circuits in the body. When I do ENERGY EXERCISES, I feel like I am hooking up these connections, so my inner system of communication will work even better!

In the same way that electrical circuits in a house can become overloaded, neurological and physiological signals can become jammed and switch off, blocking the normal flow of brain-body communication. Both Western and Eastern medical authorities recognize the need to keep the electromagnetic circuits of the body (described as meridians in the Chinese system of acupuncture) flowing freely.

During periods of increased stress, as adrenalin levels rise, a lowering of electrical potential across the nerve membrane occurs, preparing the body for fight or flight. In this state, the body reacts in order to survive, focusing electrical energy away from the neocortex and to the sympathetic nervous system. Energy Exercises and Deepening Attitudes activate the neocortex, thus refocusing electrical energy back to the reasoning centers. This stimulates parasympathetic function and decreases the release of adrenalin. By increasing the electrical threshold across the nerve membrane, thought and action are again coordinated.

Additionally, the semicircular canals of the inner ear are stimulated by electrical activity that occurs during movement. These canals, in turn, activate the brainstem's reticular formation, which screens distracting from relevant information and creates wakefulness, facilitating focus and attention in the rational centers of the brain. When the semicircular canals have been damaged or if they are not adequately stimulated by movement, a person may have difficulty concentrating. Energy Exercises and Deepening Attitudes provide a balanced stimulus to the semicircular canals, thus activating and focusing the higher brain centers for fine-motor skills and new learning.

Some of the Energy Exercises and Deepening Attitudes are derived from acupressure systems, such as Jin Shin Jitsu and Jin Shin Do. Others were inspired by Touch for Health and Applied Kinesiology techniques. Dr. Dennison combined these exercises with eye movements that enhance the sense of directionality and build visual skills on a kinesthetic basis. He gave playful names to each of the activities while working with students at his reading centers.

WATER

Water is an excellent conductor of electrical energy. Two-thirds of the human body (about seventy percent) is made up of water. All of the electrical and chemical actions of the brain and central nervous system are dependent on the conductivity of electrical currents between the brain and the sensory organs, facilitated by water. Like rain falling on the ground, water is best absorbed by the body when provided in frequent small amounts.

TEACHING TIPS

- Psychological or environmental stress depletes the body of water, leaving cells dehydrated.
- Water is essential to proper lymphatic function. (The nourishment of the cells and removal of waste is dependent on this lymphatic action.)
- All other liquids are processed in the body as food, and do not serve the body's water needs.
- Water is most easily absorbed at room temperature.
- Excessive water taken less than twenty minutes before or one hour after meals may dilute digestive juices.
- Foods that naturally contain water, like fruits and vegetables, help to lubricate the system, including the intestines. Their cleansing action facilitates absorption of water through the intestinal wall.
- Processed foods do not contain water, and, like caffeinated drinks, may be dehydrating.
- Working with electronic equipment (e.g., computer terminals, TV) is dehydrating to the body.
- The traditional way of determining water needs is to figure one ounce of water per day for every three pounds of body weight; double that in times of stress (see box).
- Unless you are a doctor, it may be illegal to prescribe water amounts for another person. With proper information, the student can determine his own needs.

ACTIVATES THE BRAIN FOR

- efficient electrical and chemical action between the brain and the nervous system
- efficient storage and retrieval of information

ACADEMIC SKILLS

- all academic skills are improved by adequate hydration
- water intake is vital before test-taking or at other times that possible stress is anticipated

BEHAVIORAL/POSTURAL CORRELATES

- improved concentration (alleviates mental fatigue)
- a heightened ability to move and participate
- improved mental and physical coordination (alleviates many difficulties related to neurological switching)
- stress release, enhancing communication and social skills

RELATED MOVEMENTS

Brain Buttons, p. 25   Hook-ups, p. 31
Earth Buttons, p. 26   Cross Crawl, p. 4
Space Buttons, p. 28

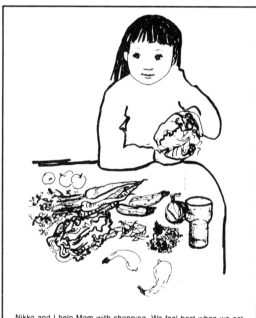

Nikko and I help Mom with shopping. We feel best when we eat foods that contain natural WATER, like fruits and vegetables, and drink plenty of good, clear WATER. In science we read that the body is made up of ⅔ WATER — a necessary conductor for all electrical and chemical reactions. More important, I know how clean and clear I feel inside, thanks to WATER!

WHY WE EMPHASIZE WATER

As a marathon runner, Dr. Dennison learned the many benefits of replenishing his system with water. At his learning centers, he noticed that students would arrive thirsty, drink great quantities of the bottled water in his office, and seem more alert and refreshed afterward. This observation led Dr. Dennison to look even further into the value of water.

Figuring Water Needs by Body Weight

weight	÷ 3	= number of ounces
# of ounces	÷ 8	= number of glasses per day
i.e., 144 lbs.	÷ 3	= 48 ounces
48 ounces	÷ 8	= 6 glasses of water per day

A 144-lb. person needs about 6 glasses of water per day.

BRAIN BUTTONS

The Brain Buttons (soft tissue under the clavicle to the left and right of the sternum) are massaged deeply with one hand while holding the navel with the other hand.

TEACHING TIPS

- The student stimulates these points for twenty to thirty seconds, or until any tenderness is released.
- The Brain Buttons may be tender at first; over a few days to a week, the tenderness subsides. Then, even holding the points will activate them.
- The student may change hands to activate both brain hemispheres.

VARIATIONS

- Include horizontal tracking (for example, across the floor or ceiling line).
- Do "Butterfly 8s" on the ceiling while holding the points: the student extends an imaginary paintbrush from his nose and paints a "Butterfly 8" on the ceiling. (Note: Butterflies are in the forward visual field, not straight overhead; the head should not be tilted back to block the "open throat" position.)
- Rather than holding the navel, massage the points to the left and right of it.

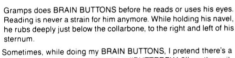

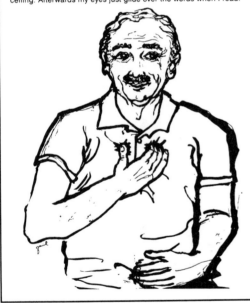

Gramps does BRAIN BUTTONS before he reads or uses his eyes. Reading is never a strain for him anymore. While holding his navel, he rubs deeply just below the collarbone, to the right and left of his sternum.

Sometimes, while doing my BRAIN BUTTONS, I pretend there's a paintbrush on my nose and paint a "BUTTERFLY 8" on the ceiling, or TRACK my eyes across the line where the wall meets the ceiling. Afterwards my eyes just glide over the words when I read.

ACTIVATE THE BRAIN FOR

- sending messages from the right brain hemisphere to the left side of the body, and vice versa
- receiving increased oxygen
- stimulation of the carotid artery for increased blood supply to the brain
- an increased flow of electromagnetic energy

ACADEMIC SKILLS

- crossing the visual midline for reading
- crossing the midline for body coordination (will facilitate an improved Cross Crawl)
- the correction of letter and number reversals
- consonant blending
- keeping one's place while reading

RELATED SKILLS

- writing, keyboard work, constructive TV or VDT watching

BEHAVIORAL/POSTURAL CORRELATES

- left-right body balance (hips not torqued, head not tilted)
- an enhanced energy level
- improved eye-teaming skills (may alleviate visual stress, squinting, or staring)
- greater relaxation of neck and shoulder muscles

RELATED MOVEMENTS

Cross Crawl, p. 4
Lazy 8s, p. 5
(See also: Earth Buttons, p. 26, Space Buttons, p. 28, Water, p. 24)

HISTORY OF THE MOVEMENT

Brain Buttons lie directly over and stimulate the carotid arteries that supply freshly oxygenated blood to the brain. The brain, though one-fiftieth of the body weight, uses one-fifth of its oxygen. Placing a hand on the navel re-establishes the gravitational center of the body, balancing the stimulus to and from the semicircular canals (centers of equilibrium in the inner ear). "Dyslexia" and related learning difficulties are associated with misinterpreted directional messages, known in Applied Kinesiology to be caused in part by visual inhibition. Brain Buttons establish a kinesthetic base for visual skills, whereby the child's ability to cross the body's lateral midline is dramatically improved.

EARTH BUTTONS

Both hands rest on the front lateral midline of the body, bringing the learner's attention to this central point of reference, necessary for making decisions regarding the positions of objects in space. When the learner can organize her visual field in terms of her own body, her eyes, hands, and whole body become better coordinated. The fingertips of one hand rest under the lower lip; the other fingertips rest at the upper edge of the pubic bone (about six inches below the navel). Experiencing this connection between the body's upper and lower halves allows the learner to coordinate them for increased stability.

TEACHING TIPS
- The points may be held for thirty seconds or more (four to six complete breaths).
- The student should breathe slowly and deeply, experiencing the relaxation.
- Instead of contacting the pubic bone, some individuals may feel more comfortable placing the palm of the lower hand over the navel, fingertips on the midline, pointing toward the ground.

VARIATIONS
- Change hands to activate both sides of the brain.
- "Zip up" the midline, without touching the body: inhale, imagining an energy fountain moving up the midline. Exhale, allowing the fountain to shower back to earth.
- Look down (for grounding) while you hold the buttons.
- Look straight down, then "walk" your vision up to a point in the distance (for near-to-far visual skills).
- Allow your eyes to track a vertical plane (e.g., ceiling to floor, at a corner).
- Rest one hand on the navel. With thumb and index finger of the other hand, lightly vibrate the points, above and below the lips, then stimulate the tailbone (a variation that combines Earth Buttons and Space Buttons).

ACTIVATE THE BRAIN FOR
- the ability to work in the midfield
- centering
- grounding (looking down to perform near-visual skills)

ACADEMIC SKILLS
- organization skills (moving eyes vertically as well as horizontally without losing one's place, as in reading columns for math or spelling)
- near-to-far visual skills (e.g., paper or book to chalkboard)
- keeping one's place while reading
- reading without disorientation

RELATED SKILLS
- organization and layout for art, bookkeeping, etc.

BEHAVIORAL/POSTURAL CORRELATES
- mental alertness (alleviates mental fatigue)
- hips level (not torqued) and head level (not tilted)
- head up and back (not slouched)
- eyes open (alleviates a squinting or staring habit)
- grounding and whole-body coordination

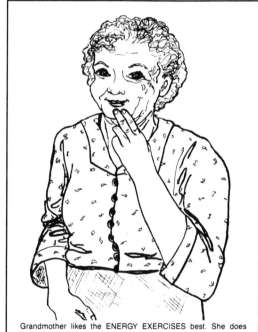

Grandmother likes the ENERGY EXERCISES best. She does EARTH BUTTONS when she balances the checkbook. "I can calculate quicker than when I was a girl back in college," she tells me, "and more precisely!" *Hold two fingers under the lower lip and rest the other hand on the upper edge of the pubic bone. Breathe the energy up the center of the body.*

RELATED MOVEMENTS
Space Buttons, p. 28   Hook-ups, p. 31
Balance Buttons, p. 27   See also: Water, p. 24

HISTORY OF THE MOVEMENT
The Earth Buttons clearly identify the lateral midline. These points are most active developmentally when the infant is learning to lift his head from a prone position or to turn from front to back, an important stage for developing binocular vision and for activating movement from the core, postural muscles outward. Touching the beginning and end points of this central acupuncture meridian also stimulates the brain, relieves mental fatigue, and makes possible the visual focus changes necessary for looking up and down.

BALANCE BUTTONS

The Balance Buttons provide a quick balance for all three dimensions: left/right, top/bottom, and back/front. Restoring balance to the occiput and the inner-ear area helps to normalize the whole body. The student holds the Balance Buttons, located just above the indentation where the skull rests over the neck (about one and one-half to two inches to each side of the back midline) and just behind the mastoid area.

TEACHING TIPS

- The student holds one Balance Button while holding the navel with the other hand for about thirty seconds, then changes hands to hold the other Balance Button. The chin is tucked in; the head is level.
- Use two or more fingers to assure that the point is covered.
- Some people may experience a pulsation when the point is stimulated or held.

VARIATIONS

- Do the activity while standing, sitting, or lying down.
- Stimulate the points by massage before holding them.
- While holding the points, draw circles around a distant object with your nose, move your head from side to side, or look all around you, relaxing both eye and neck muscles.
- Press your head gently back into your fingers while holding the points, releasing neck tension or headache.

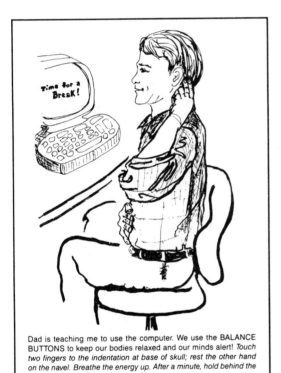

Dad is teaching me to use the computer. We use the BALANCE BUTTONS to keep our bodies relaxed and our minds alert! *Touch two fingers to the indentation at base of skull; rest the other hand on the navel. Breathe the energy up. After a minute, hold behind the other ear.*

ACTIVATE THE BRAIN FOR

- alertness and focus by stimulating the semicircular canals and reticular system
- decision-making, concentrating, and associative thinking
- changing visual focus from point to point
- increased proprioception for balance and equilibrium
- relaxed jaw and cranial movement

ACADEMIC SKILLS

- comprehension for "reading between the lines"
- perception of the author's point of view
- critical judgment and decision-making
- recognition skills for spelling and math

RELATED SKILLS

- report writing, reference work, phone or computer work
- release of motion sickness or of ear pressure built up at altitudes

BEHAVIORAL/POSTURAL CORRELATES

- a sense of well-being
- an open and receptive attitude
- eyes, ears, and head more level on shoulders
- relaxation of an overfocused posture or attitude
- improved reflexes, including Cross Crawl ability

RELATED MOVEMENTS

Positive Points, p. 32   Space Buttons, p. 28
Hook-ups, p. 31   Earth Buttons, p. 36

HISTORY OF THE MOVEMENT

When Richard H. Tyler, Doctor of Chiropractic, and Dr. Dennison did their research with students at the Valley Remedial Group Learning Center, Dr. Tyler taught the students that the Balance Buttons work to release deep levels of back-to-front switching related to weak neck muscles, long-term stress, or a head injury. Dr. Dennison later recognized this syndrome as part of the tendon-guard survival reflex, which prevents us from fully participating either expressively or receptively, especially in the area of language. When the neck muscles are strong and there is fully developed head and body differentiation, the neurological circuitry between brain and body is available for optimal performance and achievement.

SPACE BUTTONS

Both hands rest on the midline of the body–one above the upper lip on the front midline, the other on the back midline just above the tailbone. In some situations, individuals may feel more comfortable holding any point on the back midline.

TEACHING TIPS

- The student breathes energy up her spine, experiencing the resultant relaxation.
- The points may be held for thirty seconds or more (four to six complete breaths).
- Changing hands helps to activate both sides of the brain.

VARIATIONS

- The upper and lower lip may be stimulated with one hand, and the tailbone with the other (a variation using Earth Buttons and Space Buttons together).
- Stimulating the points with firm pressure or massage may be helpful, especially when tailbone falls have made sitting uncomfortable.
- Look up, or allow the eyes to track a vertical plane (e.g., ceiling to floor, at a corner) to increase visual flexibility.

ACTIVATE THE BRAIN FOR

- ability to work in the midfield
- centering and grounding
- relaxation of the central nervous system
- depth perception and visual contexts
- steadier eye contact
- near-to-far vision

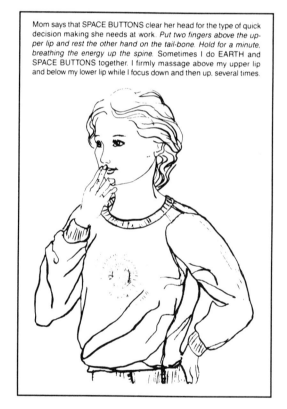

Mom says that SPACE BUTTONS clear her head for the type of quick decision making she needs at work. *Put two fingers above the upper lip and rest the other hand on the tail-bone. Hold for a minute, breathing the energy up the spine.* Sometimes I do EARTH and SPACE BUTTONS together. *I firmly massage above my upper lip and below my lower lip while I focus down and then up,* several times.

ACADEMIC SKILLS

- organization skills (moving eyes vertically as well as horizontally without confusion, as in columns for math or spelling)
- keeping one's place while reading
- the ability to focus on a task
- increased interest and motivation

RELATED SKILLS

- organization and layout for art, design, bookkeeping, or computer work

BEHAVIORAL/POSTURAL CORRELATES

- the ability to replace trying with intuition and knowing
- the ability to relax
- hips level (not torqued)
- head level (not tilted or forward)
- the ability to sit comfortably and squarely on a chair
- an increased attention span (focus alleviates hyperactive behavior)

RELATED MOVEMENTS

Earth Buttons, p. 26
Balance Buttons, p. 27
See also: Water, p. 24

HISTORY OF THE MOVEMENT

The Space Buttons are at the beginning and end points of acupuncture's governing meridian, associated with the brain, spinal column, and central nervous system. When stimulated, they facilitate increased nourishment to the brain through the blood and cerebrospinal fluid, nourishment necessary for relaxed, optimal functioning. These points are stimulated in infancy when the baby turns from back to front or is held while nursing. Space Buttons activate midlines related to all three dimensions of the body.

THE ENERGY YAWN

Yawning is a natural respiratory reflex that increases circulation to the brain and stimulates the whole body. Ideally, we should cover a yawn but avoid stifling it, which can create jaw tension. Yawning is good manners at the Brain Gym! Yawning while holding tense points on the jaw helps balance the cranial bones and relaxes tension in the head and jaw.

TEACHING TIPS

- While pretending to yawn, close eyes tight and massage the areas covering the upper and lower back molars. The muscle felt near the upper molars is involved in opening the mouth; the one felt over the lower molars does the closing of it.
- A deep, relaxed yawning sound is made while massaging the muscles.
- Repeat the activity three to six times.

VARIATIONS

- The student finds the jaw joints by opening and closing the mouth and feeling the joints with his fingertips; the mouth is comfortably opened and the student pretends to yawn while lightly massaging the muscles in front of the joint.
- Lightly hold both jaw joints, cradling the lower jaw in your palms. With relaxed mouth slightly open, ever so slowly glide your hands downward over the jaw, feeling the muscles "melt" beneath your fingers.
- To strengthen the tongue, spread it like a blanket over the upper palate while doing the Energy Yawn.

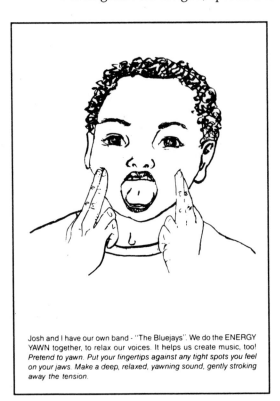

Josh and I have our own band - "The Bluejays". We do the ENERGY YAWN together, to relax our voices. It helps us create music, too! *Pretend to yawn. Put your fingertips against any tight spots you feel on your jaws. Make a deep, relaxed, yawning sound, gently stroking away the tension.*

ACTIVATES THE BRAIN FOR

- increased sensory perception and motor function of eyes and muscles for vocalization and mastication
- increased oxidation for efficient, relaxed functioning
- improved visual attention and perception
- relaxed movement of facial muscles
- enhanced verbal and expressive communication
- increased discrimination of relevant from distracting information

ACADEMIC SKILLS

- reading aloud
- creative writing
- public speaking

RELATED SKILLS

- relaxed vision and thinking during mental work
- enhanced singing

BEHAVIORAL/POSTURAL CORRELATES

- deeper vocal resonance
- relaxed vision (stimulates lubrication of the eyes)
- improved expression and creativity
- improved balance

RELATED MOVEMENTS

Cross Crawl, p. 4   The Calf Pump, p. 20
Neck Rolls, pp. 9-10   The Footflex, p. 19
Belly Breathing, p. 12

HISTORY OF THE MOVEMENT

More than fifty percent of the neurological connections between brain and body pass through the area of the jaw joint. The relationship among proprioceptors in the jaw, hips, and feet is the key to whole-body balance and equilibrium. The jaw muscles can be the most tense muscles in the body. In 1981 Dr. Dennison learned from Dr. Janet Goodrich, author of *Natural Vision Improvement*, how to yawn intentionally to improve vision. When his own eyesight improved, he added jaw-muscle massage to enhance results, and began teaching it to his students.

THE THINKING CAP

This activity helps the student focus attention on his hearing. It also relaxes tension in the cranial bones. The student uses his thumbs and index fingers to pull the ears gently back and unroll them. He begins at the top of the ear and gently massages down and around the curve, ending with the bottom lobe.

TEACHING TIPS

- The student keeps his head upright, chin comfortably level.
- The process may be repeated three or more times.

VARIATIONS

- Do the Thinking Cap in conjunction with the Energy Yawn.
- Include sounds (e.g., yawning sounds or vowel sounds).
- Do the movement while looking over a spelling list.

ACTIVATES THE BRAIN FOR

- crossing the auditory midline (including auditory recognition, attention, discrimination, perception, memory)
- listening to one's own speaking voice
- short-term working memory
- silent speech and thinking skills
- increased mental and physical fitness
- hearing with both ears together
- switched-on reticular formation (screens out distracting sounds from relevant ones)

ACADEMIC SKILLS

- listening comprehension
- public speaking, singing, playing a musical instrument
- inner speech and verbal mediation
- spelling (decoding and encoding)

RELATED SKILLS

- mental arithmetic
- concentration while working with a computer or other electronic device

BEHAVIORAL/POSTURAL CORRELATES

- improved breathing and energy
- increased voice resonance
- relaxed jaw, tongue, and facial muscles
- improved left-and-right head-turning ability
- enhanced focusing of the attention
- improved equilibrium, especially in a moving vehicle
- a better range of hearing
- expanded peripheral vision

"Let's put on our THINKING CAPS, Josh!" I remind him. (Sometimes he gets distracted and doesn't listen to what I'm saying). I put mine on too, because it helps me hear the resonant sound of my own voice when I talk or sing. *Gently unroll your ears, three times from top to bottom.*

RELATED MOVEMENTS

The Elephant, p. 8   See also: The Energy Yawn, for jaw or facial tension, p. 29
The Owl, p. 17   Water, p. 24

HISTORY OF THE MOVEMENT

This auricular exercise, used in Touch for Health, Applied Kinesiology, and acupressure systems, stimulates over 400 acupuncture points in the ears. These points are related to every function of the brain and body. Dr. Dennison discovered this activity to be particularly effective in the integration of speech and language. The Thinking Cap stimulates the reticular formation of the brain to tune out distracting, irrelevant sounds and tune in to language or other meaningful sounds. With the Thinking Cap, the meanings of words are more immediately accessible. Rhythm, sound, and imagery are simultaneously comprehended.

NOTE: For some people, excessive exposure to electronic sounds (e.g., headphones, radio, TV, a computer, video games) will switch off the ears.

HOOK-UPS

Hook-ups connect the electrical circuits in the body, containing and thus focusing both attention and disorganized energy. The mind and body relax as energy circulates through areas blocked by tension. The figure 8 pattern of the arms and legs (Part One) follows the energy flow lines of the body. The touching of the fingertips (Part Two) balances and connects the two brain hemispheres.

TEACHING TIPS

- Part One: Sitting, the student crosses the left ankle over the right. He extends his arms before him, crossing the left wrist over the right. He then interlaces his fingers and draws his hands up toward his chest. He may now close his eyes, breathe deeply, and relax for about a minute. Optional: He presses his tongue flat against the roof of his mouth on inhalation, and relaxes the tongue on exhalation.
- Part Two: When ready, the student uncrosses his legs. He touches the fingertips of both hands together, continuing to breathe deeply for about another minute.

VARIATIONS

- Hook-ups may also be done while standing.
- Cook's Hook-ups, Part 1: The student sits resting his left ankle on his right knee. He grasps his left ankle with his right hand, putting his left hand around the ball of the left foot (or shoe). He breathes deeply for about a minute, then continues with Part Two, as above.

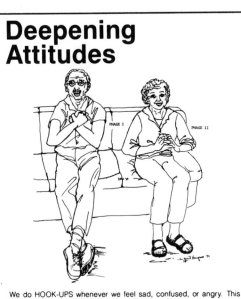

Deepening Attitudes

We do HOOK-UPS whenever we feel sad, confused, or angry. This cheers us up in no time. The activity is done in two parts. Grandpa is doing part 1. Grandma is doing part 2. *First, put your left ankle over the right one. Next, extend your arms and cross the left wrist over the right; then interlace your fingers and draw your hands up toward your chest. (Some people will feel better with the right ankle and right wrist on top.) Sit this way for one minute, breathing deeply, with your eyes closed and your tongue on the roof of your mouth. During the second part, uncross your legs and put your fingertips together, continuing to breathe deeply for another minute.*

- For Part One of any of the above versions, some people may prefer to place the right ankle and right wrist on top.

ACTIVATE THE BRAIN FOR

- emotional centering
- grounding
- increased attention (stimulates reticular formation)
- cranial movement

ACADEMIC SKILLS

- clear listening and speaking
- test-taking and similar challenges
- work at the keyboard

BEHAVIORAL/POSTURAL CORRELATES

- improved self-control and sense of boundaries
- improved balance and coordination
- increased comfort in the environment (less hypersensitivity)
- deeper respiration

RELATED MOVEMENTS

Positive Points, p. 32   Cross Crawl, p. 4
Balance Buttons, p. 27   Cross Crawl Sit-ups, p. 13

HISTORY OF THE MOVEMENT

Hook-ups shift electrical energy from the survival centers in the hindbrain to the reasoning centers in the midbrain and neocortex, thus activating hemispheric integration, increasing fine-motor coordination, and enhancing formal reasoning. Developmentally, such integration pathways are usually established in infancy through sucking and cross-motor movement. The tongue pressing into the roof of the mouth stimulates the limbic system for emotional processing in concert with more refined reasoning in the frontal lobes. Excessive energy to the receptive (right or hind) brain can manifest as depression, pain, fatigue, or hyperactivity. This energy gets redirected in Part One to the expressive (left) brain in a figure-8 pattern. Dr. Dennison discovered that this posture could also be used to release emotional stress and alleviate learning difficulties. Wayne Cook, an expert in electromagnetic energy, invented the variation of this posture (see above), from which Hook-ups are adapted, as a way to counterbalance the negative effects of electrical pollution.

POSITIVE POINTS

The student lightly touches the point above each eye with the fingertips of each hand. The points are on the frontal eminences as illustrated, halfway between the hairline and the eyebrows.

TEACHING TIPS

- The student thinks of something he would like to remember, such as the spelling of a word, or concentrates on a potentially stress-producing situation, such as a spelling test.
- The learner closes his eyes and allows himself to experience the image, or to experience the associated tension and then its release.

VARIATIONS

- Positive Points may be done in teams, one student helping the other, as illustrated.
- Positive Points may be used in conjunction with creative visualizations, such as imagining a pleasant scene, or creative thinking, such as imagining alternative outcomes to an event or story.
- Positive Points may be gently massaged to relieve visual stress.

ACTIVATE THE BRAIN FOR

- accessing the frontal lobe to balance stress around specific memories, situations, people, places, and skills
- relaxing the reflex to act without thinking when under stress

ACADEMIC SKILLS

- the release of memory blocks (e.g., "I know the answer. It's on the tip of my tongue.")
- useful when studying spelling, mathematics, and social studies, or whenever long-term memory is required

RELATED SKILLS

- sports performance
- public speaking
- stage performance
- reading aloud

BEHAVIORAL/POSTURAL CORRELATES

- organizational abilities
- study skills
- test performance

RELATED MOVEMENTS

Water, p. 24
Hook-ups, p. 31
Belly Breathing, p. 12
Think of an X, p. 15

I am holding my Dad's POSITIVE POINTS. We hold these points for ourselves or for each other whenever we feel nervous or afraid. We know we can achieve our goals when we stop worrying about things and start working on them. In less than a minute, we begin to feel peaceful about planning for the future. *The positive points are held lightly, with just enough pressure to pull the forehead skin taut. The points are just above the eyeballs, halfway between the hairline and the eyebrow.*

HISTORY OF THE MOVEMENT

The Dennisons renamed these emotional-stress release points from Touch for Health "the Positive Points." These points are the neurovascular balance points for the stomach meridian. People tend to hold stress in the abdomen, resulting in stomachaches and nervous stomachs, a pattern often established in early childhood while sophisticated cortical development is taking place. The Positive Points bring blood flow from the hypothalamus to the frontal lobes, where rational thought occurs. This prevents the fight-or-flight response, so that a new response to the situation can be learned.

Brain Gym at Work...and Play!

READING SKILLS

Crossing the Visual Midline

Moving the eyes across the page without inhibiting the receptive brain

The development of visual skills for reading begins with the ability to move both eyes in tandem from left to right across the midline of the page and across the corresponding visual midfield. For reading, one eye must be dominant for focusing, the other eye for blending. Although both skills are available to each eye, stress in learning the tasks of focusing and blending for reading may cause visual disorientation.

Brain Buttons - p. 25
Cross Crawl - p. 4
Lazy 8's - p. 5
Butterfly - p. 25
Tracking - p. 25

Smooth Reading across the Midline

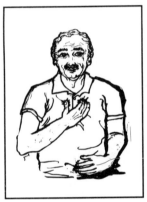

Brain Buttons

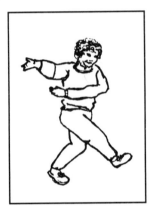

Cross Crawl

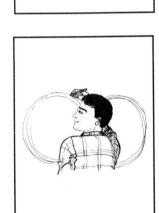

Lazy 8s

Oral Reading

Expressive reading with emotion and interpretation

The reader must discover that he or she is telling a story and communicating ideas through reading. One must have the concept of a verbal code in order for true reading to be possible. In Western languages, the code includes an auditory as well as a visual and a motor component. All three of these must be used together for reconstruction of the code to take place.

Reading Aloud

Neck Rolls - p. 9
Energy Yawn - p. 29
Cross Crawl - p. 4
Rocker - p. 11
Belly Breathing - p. 12

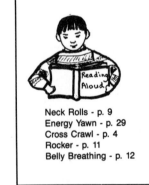

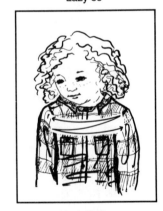

Neck Rolls

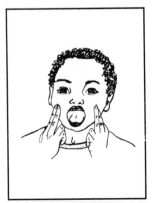

The Energy Yawn

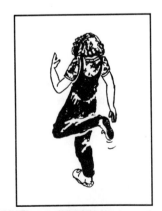

Cross Crawl

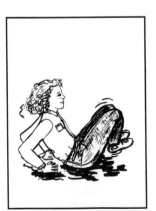

The Rocker

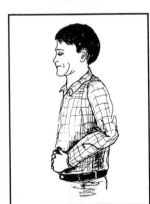

Belly Breathing

Reading Comprehension

Focused reading involving anticipation and internalization of language

Reading is an active reconstruction by the reader of the author's message or code. There's nothing inherently meaningful about the code itself. The success of the communication depends upon the writer encoding something meaningful and the reader decoding it, making it his or her own. Thus, communication through the written word depends on the reader's active recreation of the work as he or she reads it.

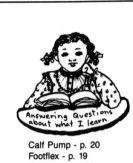

Calf Pump - p. 20
Footflex - p. 19
Grounder - p. 22

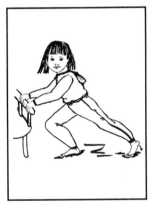

The Calf Pump

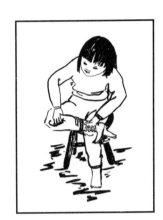

The Footflex

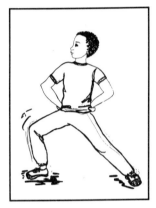

The Grounder

THINKING SKILLS

Organization Skills

Moving the eyes vertically as well as horizontally without confusion

Familiarity with multimodality (visual, auditory, tactile, kinesthetic) and multidirectional processes is a prerequisite for comprehending math and spelling. Until left, right, up, and down are recognized as unique visual spaces, the learner will have difficulty with words or symbols presented in columns, and with placing symbols in an ordered sequence.

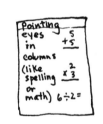

Earth Buttons - p.26
Space Buttons - p.28
Balance Buttons - p.27

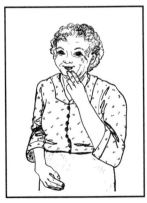

Earth Buttons

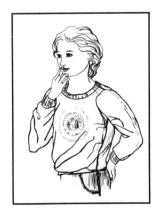

Space Buttons

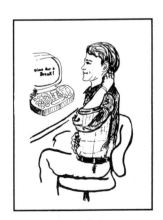

Balance Buttons

Spelling

The ability to access visual memory and simultaneously build auditory constructs

For efficient spelling, development of both short- and long-term memory for storage of information about sounds and associations is essential.

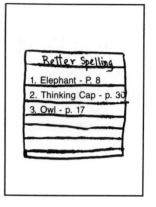

Better Spelling
1. Elephant - P. 8
2. Thinking Cap - p. 30
3. Owl - p. 17

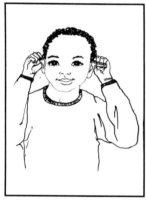

The Thinking Cap

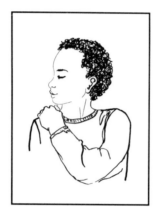

The Owl

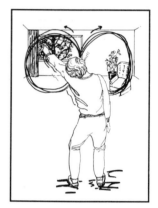

The Elephant

Math

The ability to work in a multidimensional, multidirectional medium

Math skills are more accessible to the student who has internalized concepts about space, mass, quantities, and relationships.

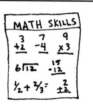

MATH SKILLS

Elephant - p. 8
The Owl - p. 17
Calf Pump - p. 20
Neck Rolls - p. 9
Gravity Glider - p. 21

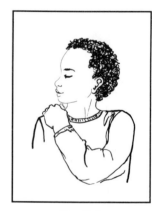

The Owl

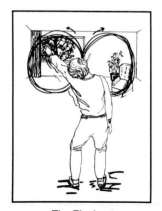

The Elephant

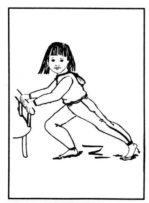

The Calf Pump

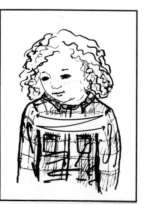

Neck Rolls

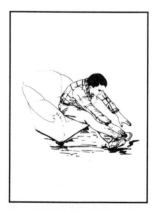

The Gravity Glider

WRITING SKILLS

Eye-Hand Coordination

Penmanship, cursive writing, and drawing in the left, right, upper, and lower visual fields

The learner discovers that symbols (letters or pictures) can communicate meaning. The desire to communicate through symbols is the first step in acquiring writing skills. Gross-motor movement is established as a basis for handedness and fine-motor control.

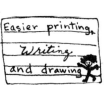

Lazy 8's - p. 5
Alphabet 8's - p. 7
Arm Activation - p. 18
Double Doodle - p. 6

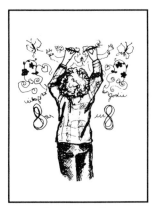

Double Doodle

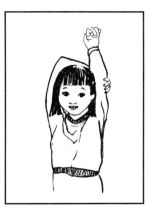

Arm Activation

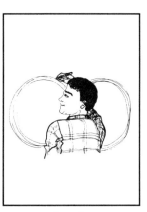

Lazy 8s

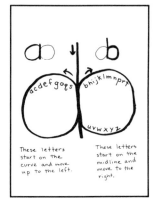

Alphabet 8s

Creative Writing

The ability to express experiences received and stored in the hindbrain as personal language

Skills of reading and writing the code develop together, each reinforcing the other. Writing helps to establish the skills of attention (focus), perception (meaning), and discrimination (connecting the code to associations and feelings). Writing skills must keep pace with reading skills, and ideally are maintained at a level no more than two years below the reading level.

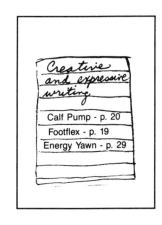

Calf Pump - p. 20
Footflex - p. 19
Energy Yawn - p. 29

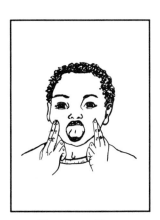

The Energy Yawn

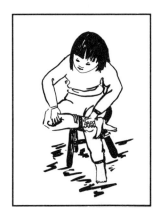

The Footflex

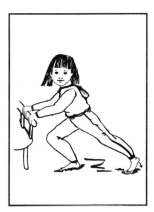

The Calf Pump

SELF-AWARENESS SKILLS

Crossing the Auditory Midline:
Clear Listening and Speaking

Active listening involves both external and internal feedback and feedforward

Active listening involves both reception and processing of meaning, and is a basic prerequisite to all effective communication. Externally, motor responses are necessary for hearing and speech. Internally, one must interpret thoughts and associations to be able to respond from one's experience. The feedback-feedforward loop allows comprehension and expression to take place.

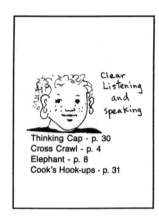

Clear Listening and speaking
Thinking Cap - p. 30
Cross Crawl - p. 4
Elephant - p. 8
Cook's Hook-ups - p. 31

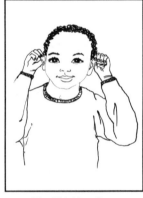

The Thinking Cap

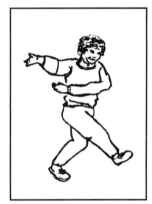

Cross Crawl

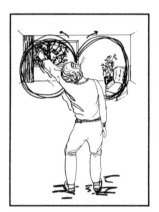

The Elephant

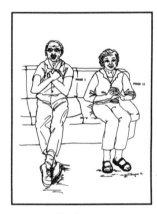

Hook-ups

Self-Concept: Inner Sunshine

Self-esteem is both the goal and the means of self-directed learning

Having confidence within the boundaries of personal space helps one to feel safe, to know when risk-taking is appropriate, and to respect other people's space. Personal space is the immediate working area around the body, including all the space one can comfortably reach in any direction. Into this space, we can radiate our thoughts, feelings, and self-expression.

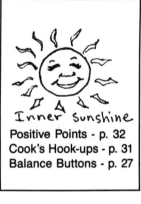

Inner sunshine
Positive Points - p. 32
Cook's Hook-ups - p. 31
Balance Buttons - p. 27

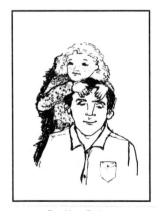

Positive Points

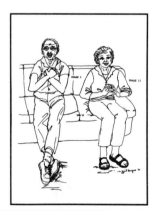

Hook-ups

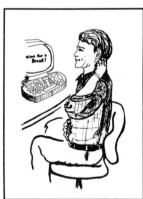

Balance Buttons

Whole-Body Coordination for Sports and Play

Basic brain-body reflexes are essential for decision-making while one is in motion

The learner develops a sense of the physical area of his personal space and defines his boundaries. This safe space has left/right, top/bottom, and back/front dimensions. Improved visual and kinesthetic figure-ground manifest on the playing field as ease of tracking and hand-eye coordination. The learner discovers greater autonomy while coordinating his brain and body through focused movement.

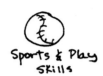

Sports & Play Skills

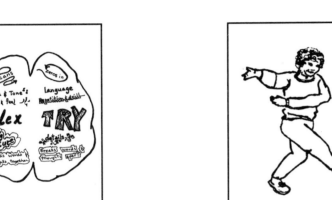

Think of an X

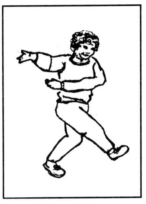

Cross Crawl

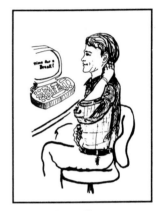

Balance Buttons

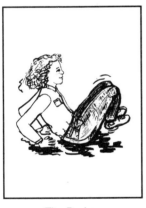

The Rocker

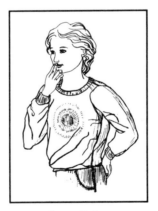

Space Buttons

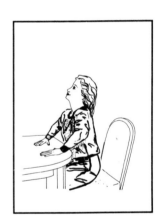

The Energizer

HOME-STUDY SKILLS

Memory and Abstract Thinking

Integration of silent speech and visualization skills, better known as thinking

Silent speech is necessary to interpret abstract concepts and to process language once reading vocabulary exceeds speaking vocabulary (sixth-grade level). Auditory and visual input must be integrated to enable the storage of information into short-term memory for analytical use and the retrieval of information from long-term memory for verbal expression.

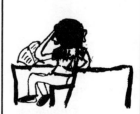

Cross Crawl - p. 4
Balance Buttons - p. 27
Positive Points - p. 32
Neck Rolls - p. 9

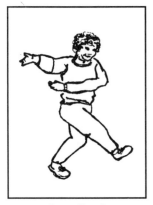

Cross Crawl

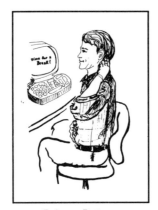

Balance Buttons

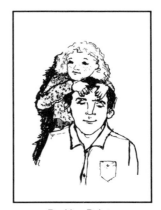

Positive Points

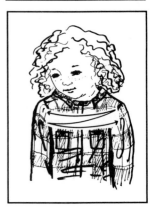

Neck Rolls

Creative Thinking

Integration of what is presented by others with one's own life and thought

Focus, attention, and concentration require integration of prior life experiences (actual, imaginary, or vicarious) and new information (received by the hindbrain and expressed in language through the forebrain), so that the new is processed and stored as personal knowledge.

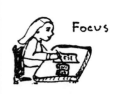

Cross Crawl - p. 4
Any Lengthening
Activities p. 16-22
The Energizer - p. 14
The Rocker - p. 11

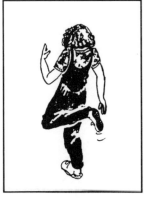

Cross Crawl

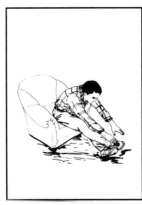

The Gravity Glider

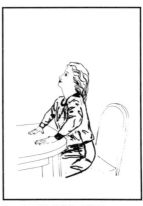

The Energizer

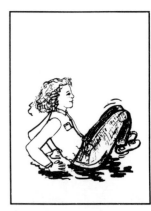

The Rocker

Speed-Reading

Skimming and scanning abilities made accessible

In speed-reading, one bypasses as much of the linear process as possible while still actively taking in information. Skimming is exploring the printed page for meaningful material, while skipping the redundant. Scanning is reviewing the data for anticipated information, such as a name or date. The skilled speed-reader varies his speed according to writing style and subject matter.

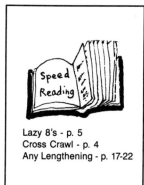

Lazy 8's - p. 5
Cross Crawl - p. 4
Any Lengthening - p. 17-22

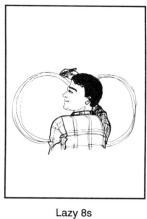

Lazy 8s

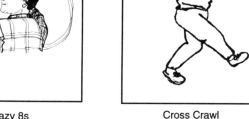

Cross Crawl

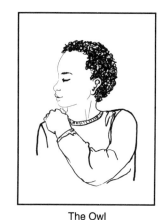

The Owl

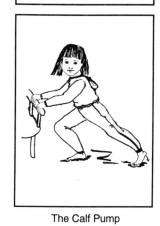

The Calf Pump

Test Taking

Relaxing the butterflies

Information which has been learned or experienced is stored in the long-term memory centers of the brain. The ability to retrieve and use this information, especially in a situation which tests our skills and abilities, requires focus and presence, without confusion, anxiety, or distraction.

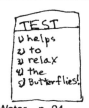

Water - p. 24
Lazy 8's - p. 5
Earth Buttons - p. 26
Space Buttons - p. 28
Cook's Hook-ups-p. 31
Cross Crawl - p. 4

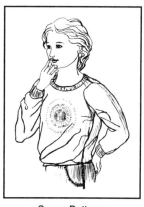

Space Buttons

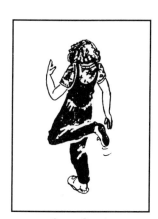

Cross Crawl

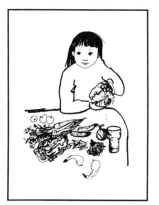

Water

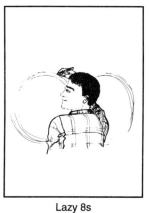

Lazy 8s

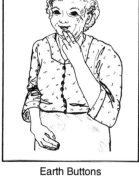

Earth Buttons

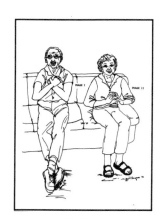

Hook-ups

PERSONAL ECOLOGY SKILLS

Productivity at the Keyboard and Video Screen

The ability to stabilize homeostasis

For the sensitive individual, electronic devices may aggravate visual, auditory, or other physiological stresses. The video screen provides only one visual plane, limiting the use of binocular vision, depth perception, and peripheral vision. The constant hum of many devices switches off auditory skills, while the electromagnetic field of radio-controlled equipment may negatively affect body meridians.

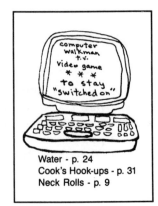

Water - p. 24
Cook's Hook-ups - p. 31
Neck Rolls - p. 9

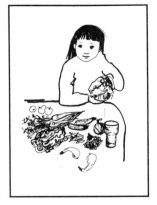

Water

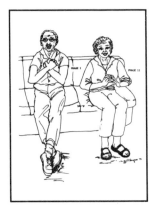

Hook-ups

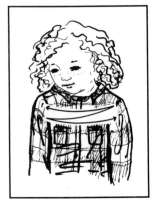

Neck Rolls

Riding in a Car, Bus, or Plane

Crossing the moving midline

The body must keep its sense of balance in a moving vehicle by compensating with the inner ear for motion left to right, back to front, or side to side. Binocular vision and depth perception may also be affected by this motion.

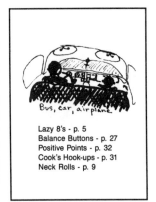

Lazy 8's - p. 5
Balance Buttons - p. 27
Positive Points - p. 32
Cook's Hook-ups - p. 31
Neck Rolls - p. 9

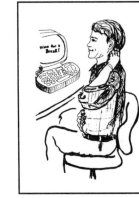

Balance Buttons

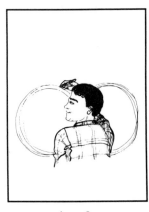

Lazy 8s

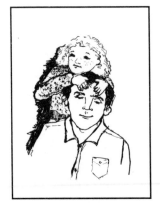

Positive Points

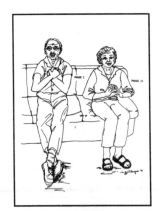

Hook-ups

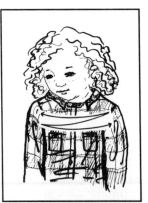

Neck Rolls

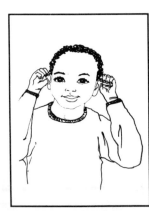

The Thinking Cap

An Overview of Experimental Research Using Brain Gym

The following is a compilation of professional publications and research abstracts from presentations at various conferences. It deals with the experimental research which has been completed using Brain Gym and other Educational Kinesiology techniques in controlled situations. Each reference is followed by a brief summary of the information contained within the longer work.

Publications

Khalsa, Guruchiter Kaur, Morris, G. S. Don, & Sifft, Josie M. (1988). Effect of Educational Kinesiology on static balance of learning-disabled students. *Perceptual and Motor Skills, 67,* 51-54.

> This publication is the short research journal report of the first experimental study conducted using Educational Kinesiology techniques. The study was conducted by Guruchiter Kaur Khalsa as a Master's thesis in the Department of Health, Physical Education, and Recreation at the California State Polytechnic University.

Khalsa, Guruchiter K. and Sifft, Josie M. (1988). *The Effects of Educational Kinesiology Upon the Static Balance of Learning-disabled Boys and Girls.* (ERIC Document Reproduction Service No. ED 289 835)

> This publication, the hard copy of a presentation made to the American Alliance for Health, Physical Education, Recreation and Dance National Convention in Las Vegas, Nevada, in April of 1987, provides detailed information on the first experimental study conducted using Educational Kinesiology techniques, including some Brain Gym activities and Dennison Laterality Repatterning. The full publication is available from Educational Resources Information Center, or can be viewed on microfiche.

Sifft, Josie M. (1990). Educational Kinesiology: Empowering Students and Athletes Through Movement. (ERIC Document Reproduction Service No. ED 320891)

> This publication, the hard copy of a presentation made to the American Alliance for Health, Physical Education, Recreation and Dance National Convention in New Orleans, Louisiana, in April of 1990, provides an overview of Educational Kinesiology, an explanation of some of the Brain Gym activities, and a report of the research to date. The full publication is available from Educational Resources Information Center, or can be viewed on microfiche.

Sifft, Josie M. and G.C.K. Khalsa (1991). Effect of Educational Kinesiology upon simple response times and choice response times. *Perceptual and Motor Skills, 73,* 1011-1015.

> This publication is the short research journal report of the second experimental study conducted using Educational Kinesiology techniques. The study was done with university students to see whether Brain Gym activities and Laterality Repatterning would influence the response times to a visual stimulus. The results indicated that both Edu-K groups were superior to the control group and that the Repatterned group improved twice as much as the Brain Gym-only group.

Research Abstracts

"Effect of Educational Kinesiology upon the Static Balance of Learning-Disabled Boys and Girls," Khalsa, Guruchiter Kaur and Sifft, Josie M. American Alliance for Health, Physical Education, Recreation and Dance National Convention, April, 1987, Las Vegas, Nevada.

> This study was completed with sixty elementary students who were classified as learning-disabled. An equal number of boys and girls were divided into three groups: Repatterned Edu-K, Edu-K movement, and a control. The results indicated that the Repatterned Edu-K group showed a greater improvement in static balance than the Edu-K movement group, who in turn performed better than the control group. The findings also suggest that Edu-K can be used effectively in a coeducational setting.

"Effect of Educational Kinesiology Upon Simple and Four-Choice Response Times," Sifft, Josie M. and Khalsa, Guruchiter Kaur. American Alliance for Health, Physical Education, Recreation and Dance Southwest District Convention, March, 1989, Salt Lake City, Utah.

> This study completed with university students compared a control group with two experimental groups, one using only Brain Gym activities and the other experiencing Dennison Laterality Repatterning and the Brain Gym activities. The results indicated that the Edu-K groups were superior to the control group in their response time to a four-choice visual light display. The repatterned group improved by twice the amount of the Brain Gym-only group.

"Effect of Educational Kinesiology on Hearing," Sifft, Josie M. and Khalsa, Guruchiter Kaur. California Association for Health, Physical Education, Recreation and Dance Regional Conference, December, 1990, Long Beach, California.

> This study was completed with sixteen elementary school teachers who served as their own control. Each teacher was tested on the Pure-tone audiometer before and after each movement experience. The movement experiences were ten minutes of random movements about the room or a series of five Brain Gym activities. The results indicated that the hearing of the teachers was better after the Brain Gym activities than after the random movements.

"Effect of Educational Kinesiology on Response Times of Learning-Disabled Students," Khalsa, Guruchiter Kaur and Sifft, Josie M., unpublished manuscript.

> This study was completed with fifty-two children selected from Special Education classes. The Brain Gym group performed a sequence of activities, while the control group engaged in random movements for about seven minutes. All children were tested for visual response time before and after the movement activities. The results indicated that those children exposed to the Brain Gym movements improved on the response time task, while those in the control group did not.

Glossary

accommodation – The rapid, automatic ability to adjust focus to fit visual needs.

analytic – Refers to the ability to perceive reality as isolated, separate parts without attention to their context as a whole.

bilaterality – The ability to coordinate two sides to function as a single unit.

binocular integration – Eye-teaming ability, essential if the two eyes and all their reciprocating muscles are to work as one.

blending – The visual or auditory synthesis of separate parts, such as syllables or phonetic speech sounds for reading, into longer, more meaningful wholes.

centering – The ability to cross the dividing line between emotional content and abstract thought; also, the organization of body reflexes.

convergence – The ability to point the two eyes so that the visual axes of both eyes lie on the image being fixated, so that binocular fusion is possible.

compensatory approach – The outmoded approach to education for learning disabilities which emphasizes that children must accept their situation and learn to adjust to it by maximizing a strength and compensating for any weaknesses.

cranial movement – The ability of the cranial bones in the skull to move during breathing, movement, and learning.

cross crawl – Any contralateral movement whereby one side of the body moves in coordination with the other side, requiring bihemispheric brain activation.

decode – The analysis of any symbolic language for translation into a meaningful message.

depth perception – The ability to see objects as three-dimensional or to judge the relative spatial distance between objects.

dominance – The inherited preference for one cerebral hemisphere over the other for handedness, eyedness, earedness, etc.

dyslexia – The label used to describe the perceived inability to decode the printed symbol due to the inhibition of the receptive centers of the brain. Broadly, any learning disability which causes confusion and compensatory behaviors.

ecology – The study of the interdependence of living and nonliving things in a closed system or environment.

Educational Kinesiology – The study of movement and its relationship to whole-brain learning.

Edu-Kinesthetics – The application of kinesthetics (movement) to the study of right-brain, left-brain, and body integration for purposes of eliminating stress and maximizing full learning potential.

encode – To express meaning and language through the use of written symbols.

eye-hand coordination – Visual-motor skill: the basis for working with any aspect of written language, including reading, spelling, and mathematics.

feedback – The short-term memory skill that enables one to hear one's voice repeating something thought, read, or heard.

feedforward – The short-term memory skill that enables one to anticipate one's voice speaking from long-term memory.

focus – The ability to concentrate on one part of one's experience, differentiating it from other parts through awareness of its similarities and differences.

fusion – The ability of the brain to blend together the information coming in from both eyes.

gestalt – The perception of reality as a whole or totality without attention to analysis of its separate parts.

homolateral – Involuntarily choosing to access only one cerebral hemisphere, blocking integrated thought and movement.

integration – The lifelong process of realizing one's physical, mental, and spiritual potential, the first step being the simultaneous activation of both cerebral hemispheres for specific learning; the act of making whole, complete.

lateral skills – Communication, language, and near-point skills that require left-to-right spatial orientation.

linear – That which is processed sequentially, over time, rather than gestalted spontaneously.

midfield – The area where a person's two visual fields overlap for integrated learning.

midline – The line that separates one visual field and hemispheric awareness from the other.

mixed dominance – (also called cross dominance) The brain-organization pattern in which one is dominant with one hand, usually the right, and dominant with the alternate eye and/or ear at the same time.

overfocus – The extreme state of attention wherein one loses the ability to see details in relation to the overall context in which they exist.

peripheral vision – The ability to be aware of information from the sides of the body while focusing straight ahead.

reflex – To act without conscious thought and with self-preservation as the primary motivation. Used as a verb in Edu-Kinesthetics to suggest the movements initiated by the gestalt brain when one is homolateral and not yet integrated.

saccadic eye movement – The movement of the eyes when one is shifting attention from one focus to another.

scanning – The ability to move the eyes about the environment to gestalt information without conscious fixation.

skimming – The ability to fixate on relevant details efficiently, screening out other visual information.

switched off – The state of involuntary inhibition of one cerebral hemisphere in order to better access the other, due to stress or lack of integration.

visual gate – The ability to be aware of a double image when focusing past the image into the distance.

Bibliography and Recommended Reading

Armstrong, Thomas, Ph.D. *In Their Own Way: Discovering and Encouraging Your Child's Personal Learning Style.* Los Angeles, CA: Jeremy P. Tarcher, Inc., 1987.

Anderson, Bob. *Stretching.* Bolinas, CA: Shelter Publications, Inc., 1980.

Ayres, A. Jean. *Sensory Integration and Learning Disorders.* Los Angeles, CA: Western Psychological Services, 1973.

Benzwie, Teresa, Ph.D. *A Moving Experience: Dance for Lovers of Children and the Child Within.* Tucson, AZ: Zephyr Press, 1987.

Brookes, Mona. *Drawing With Children.* Los Angeles, CA: Jeremy P. Tarcher, Inc., 1986.

Buzan, Tony. *Use Both Sides of Your Brain.* New York, NY: E.P. Dutton, 1974.

Canfield, Jack and Wells, Harold. *100 Ways to Enhance Self-Concept in the Classroom.* Englewood Cliffs, NJ: Prentice Hall, Inc., 1976.

Cherry, Clare; Goodwin, Douglas; Staples, Jesse. *Is the Left Brain Always Right?* Belmont, CA: Fearon Teacher Aids, 1989.

Clark, Linda. *Optimizing Learining: The Integrative Education Model in the Classroom.* Columbus, OH: Merill Publishing Company, 1986.

Cobb, Vicki. *How to Really Fool Yourself (Illustrations for All Your Senses).* New York, NY: J.B. Lippincott, 1981.

Delacato, Carl H. *The Diagnosis and Treatment of Speech and Reading Problems.* Springfield, IL: Charles C. Thomas, 1963.

Dennison. (See book list at front of book.)

Gardner, Howard. *Frames of Mind: The Theory of Multiple Intelligences.* New York, NY: Basic Books, Inc., 1985.

Getman, Gerald N., O.D., D.O.S., *How to Develop Your Child's Intelligence.* Irvine, CA: Research Publications, 1984.

_____ *Smart in Everything . . . Except School.* Santa Ana, CA: VisionExtension, Inc., 1992.

Gilbert, Ann Green. *Teaching the Three Rs Through Movement Experiences.* New York, NY: Macmillan Publishing Co., 1977.

Goodrich, Janet. *Natural Vision Improvement.* Berkeley, CA: Celestial Arts, 1986.

Kavner, Richard S., O.D. *Your Child's Vision.* New York, NY: Kavner Books, 1985.

Kephart, Newell C. *The Slow Learner in the Classroom.* Columbus, OH: Charles C. Merrill, 1960.

Lyman, Donald E. *Making the Words Stand Still.* Boston, MA: Houghton Mifflin Co., 1986.

Mander, Jerry. *Four Arguments for the Elimination of Television.* New York, NY: William Morrow and Company, Inc., 1978.

Montessori, Maria. *The Absorbent Mind.* New York, NY: Rinehart, 1967.

Ostrander, S. and Schroeder, L. *Superlearning.* New York, NY: Dell Publishing Co., Inc., 1979.

Ott, John. *Health and Light.* Old Greenwich, CT: The Devin-Adair Co., 1973.

Pearce, Joseph Chilton. *The Magical Child Matures.* New York, NY: Bantam Books, 1986.

Pelletier, Kenneth R. *Mind as Healer, Mind as Slayer.* New York, NY: Delta Press, 1977.

Spache, G.B., Hinds, L.R., Ging, L.B., et al. *Vision and School Success.* Cleveland, OH: Clarion, 1990.

Thie, John F., D.C. *Touch for Health.* Marina del Rey, CA: DeVorss & Co., 1973.

Walthers, David S. *Applied Kinesiology: The Advanced Approach to Chiropractic.* Pueblo, CO: Systems DC, 1976.

Weiner, Harold. *Eyes OK, I'm OK.* San Raphael, CA: Academic Therapy Publications, 1977.

For more information on optometric vision research and training, contact: Optometric Extension Program Foundation, Inc., 2912 South Daimler Street, Suite 100, Santa Ana, CA 92705-5811, (714) 250-0846.